Case Studies in Neurosurgery for the House Officer

D0873394

Case Studies in Neurosurgery for the House Officer

Robert A. Solomon, MD

Assistant Professor
Neurological Surgery

Michael B. Sisti, MD

Resident of Neurological Surgery

Department of Neurological Surgery
The Neurological Institute of New York
Columbia—Presbyterian Medical Center
Columbia University College of Physicians and Surgeons
New York, New York

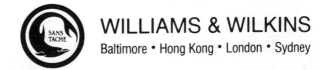

WILLIAMS & WILKINS

Baltimore • Hong Kong • London • Sydney

Editor: Kimberly Kist
Associate Editor: Victoria M. Vaughn
Copy Editor: Susan Vaupel
Design: Dan Pfisterer
Illustration Planning: Lorraine Wrzosek
Production: Charles E. Zeller

Accurate indications, adverse reactions, and dosage schedules for drugs are provided in this book, but it is possible that they may change. The reader is urged to review the package information data of the manufacturers of the medications mentioned.

Printed in the United States of America

Library of Congress Cataloging in Publication Data

Case studies in neurosurgery for the house officer / [edited by]
    Robert A. Solomon, Michael B. Sisti; contributing authors, Paul McCormick . . . [et al.].
    p.   cm.
    Includes index.
    ISBN 0-683-07858-5
    1. Neurology — Case   Studies.   2. Nervous   system — Surgery — Case   studies.
I. Solomon, Robert A.   II. Sisti, Michael B.   III. McCormick, Paul, 1956–
    [DNLM: 1. Brain Injuries—diagnosis—case studies. 2. Nervous System Diseases—
diagnosis—case studies.   WL 141 C337]
    RC359.C37 1989
    616.8'049—dc19
    DNLM/DLC
    for Library of Congress   88-26187
                                                                              CIP

89   90   91   92   10   9   8   7   6   5   4   3   2

Series Editor's Foreword

The series, Case Studies for the House Officer, has been designed to teach medicine by a case study approach. It is considered a supplement to the parent House Officer Series which provides information in a problem-oriented format. *Neurosurgery for the House Officer* has proved popular with house officers and medical students. In *Case Studies in Neurosurgery for the House Officer*, Doctors Solomon, Sisti, and their colleagues at Columbia have compiled an impressive series of interesting cases that cover the most common neurosurgical problems. They have added thoughtful "Pearls" and "Pitfalls" and pertinent x-rays, CT scans, or MRIs. The book should be a useful and enjoyable learning experience for students of neurosurgery.

Lawrence P. Levitt, M.D.
Senior Consultant in Neurology
Lehigh Valley Hospital Center
Allentown, Pennsylvania
Clinical Professor of Neurology
Hahnemann University and Clinical Associate Professor
Temple University School of Medicine

Preface

Case Studies in Neurosurgery for the House Officer
is a book that grew from the busy clinical service of
the Department of Neurological Surgery at the
Neurological Institute of Columbia Presbyterian
Medical Center in New York. This book is meant to be
a guide for neurosurgical house officers and medical
students. The entire resident staff of the
Neurological Institute was invited to participate in
the development of this collection of instructive
cases. The goal was to collect a series of diverse
cases which as a whole would constitute a
representative sampling of the great majority of
problems encountered in clinical neurosurgery. No
attempt has been made to give a detailed or
exhaustive discussion of individual topics, instead
the reader is instructed to consult the key
references that are listed at the end of each
chapter. This book is not meant to be a text of
neurosurgery, instead it should serve as a means of
self-assessment for the neurosurgical house officer
and an enjoyable introduction into the clinical side
of neurosurgery for the medical students and surgical
interns rotating on neurosurgery services.

Acknowledgment

This manual was edited and typed for publication by Regina Ann Hartley. The Department of Neurological Surgery is grateful to her for the secretarial preparation of this manuscript.

Contributors

Paul McCormick, MD
Robert Goodman, MD
Jeffrey Bruce, MD
Karin Muraszko, MD
Charles Reidel, MD
Dale Swift, MD
Joseph Alexander, MD
Jon Grant, MD
Stephen Onesti, MD
Michel Kliot, MD

Department of Neurological Surgery
The Neurological Institute of New York
Columbia—Presbyterian Medical Center
Columbia University College of Physicians and Surgeons
New York, New York

Contents

UNILATERAL TINNITUS AND HEARING LOSS

CASE 1: This 58-year-old woman was well except for a 2-month history of tinnitus in the right ear. When she consulted her physician about this problem, it was noted that she had dramatically reduced hearing in the right ear. The neurological exam was otherwise normal and a CT scan was performed.

Clue: CT scan of patient.

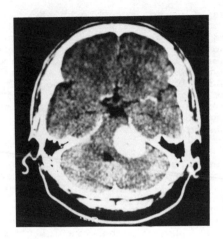

Figure 1.1

QUESTIONS:

1. What is the diagnosis in this case?

2. Which cranial nerves are involved by this tumor?

3. What are the goals of surgical treatment for this patient?

4. Describe two different surgical approaches to this lesion. What are the benefits and drawbacks of each?

5. What types of special intraoperative monitoring might be useful for this case?

ANSWERS:

1. A <u>schwannoma of the VIIIth nerve (acoustic neuroma)</u>
    is the most common tumor to present in the
    cerebellopontine angle. The classic neurological
    presentation and the CT appearance confirm this
    diagnosis.

2. <u>Three cranial nerves run through the
    cerebellopontine angle: facial nerve, cochlear
    nerve, and vestibular nerve</u>. Acoustic neuromas
    most commonly originate from the vestibular nerve,
    one of the two components of the VIIIth cranial
    nerve. Symptoms from this tumor are most often
    referable to compression of the cochlear nerve with
    consequent hearing loss and tinnitus. It is rare
    for acoustic neuromas to produce symptoms referable
    to the vestibular nerve or the facial nerve, even
    though these nerves are often severely deformed by
    the tumor.

3. The goal of surgical therapy in this case is <u>total
    extirpation of the tumor</u> with preservation of the
    VIIth and VIIIth nerve function. Modern
    microsurgical techniques have allowed surgeons to
    remove even large tumors in this location without
    anatomical disruption of the VIIth nerve. The
    VIIIth nerve appears to be more delicate than the
    VIIth nerve and therefore it is more difficult to
    preserve hearing than facial function when acoustic
    neuromas are removed. However, with small tumors
    that are diagnosed with hearing still intact,
    preservation of the VIIIth nerve should be
    attempted.

4. Two different operations have been widely used to
    remove acoustic neuromas: a translabyrinthine
    approach and the more traditional suboccipital
    posterior fossa approach. The <u>translabyrinthine
    operation involves a dissection through the
    external ear, and the facial nerve is encountered
    before the tumor</u>. Some surgeons feel that facial
    nerve preservation is facilitated by this approach
    because the nerve can be identified early in the

procedure. The disadvantages are that this
approach is only useful for small tumors, and
hearing must be sacrificed as the labyrinth is
opened.

The suboccipital approach allows for the
possibility that hearing can be preserved. This
approach is safer for large tumors as the brain
stem and vascular structures of the posterior fossa
can be well visualized and protected during the
operation. The entire extent of the tumor can be
appreciated from the suboccipital approach, whereas
the visualization is not nearly as good in the
translabyrinthine operation. The major drawback of
the suboccipital approach is that the risk of
serious morbidity and mortality is relatively
greater, because the posterior fossa is opened and
the cerebellum must be retracted.

5. Technological advances in intraoperative
   monitoring have greatly facilitated the safe
   surgical removal of acoustic neuromas. Techniques
   can be utilized to provide continuous feedback to
   the surgeon as to the functional integrity of
   cranial nerves and the brain stem.

   Facial nerve stimulation is useful in
   identifying the nerve and periodically assessing
   its function. The most elegant way of monitoring
   facial muscular response to stimulation is with
   electromyograph (EMG). EMG eliminates the need for
   direct visualization of the face during the
   operation, and impulses can be detected not only
   when the nerve is stimulated, but also when the
   nerve is retracted or threatened during dissection.

   Brain stem auditory evoked responses (BAERs) are
   extremely valuable. Repetitive "clicking" sounds
   are constantly delivered to the ear and the
   resulting potentials that appear in the cortical
   electrocephalogram (EEG) are computer averaged to
   subtract the background activity. Recordings of
   these potentials provide information not only about
   the integrity of the brain stem, but also the
   functional state of the eighth nerve.

PEARLS:

1. The anatomy of the nerves that run through the
    porous acousticus is vitally important to the
    neurosurgeon's effort to save the facial and
    auditory nerves. As the VIIth and VIIIth cranial
    nerves leave the brain stem, the VIIth nerve is
    ventral to the VIIIth nerve elements. However, as
    the nerves cross the cerebellar pontine angle to
    reach the internal auditory meatus, they rotate 90°
    so that the facial nerve is situated anterior and
    superior, the auditory nerve is anterior and
    inferior, and the vestibular nerves run
    posteriorly. This configuration accounts for the
    fact that the facial nerve most often sweeps around
    the anterior border of the tumor, because these
    tumors arise from the vestibular component of the
    VIIIth nerve as it enters the internal auditory
    meatus.

2. Very tiny, often insignificant appearing arterial
    twigs frequently constitute the primary blood
    supply to the cochlea and the auditory nerve.
    Irreversible hearing loss can be produced by
    disruption of these tiny vessels. Therefore, when
    preservation of hearing is an important goal of the
    operation, the surgeon must be careful to spare the
    small arteries that travel with the
    vestibulocochlear nerves, and avoid excessive
    cautery.

3. Acoustic neuromas are occasionally found in
    patients with von Recklinghausen's
    neurofibromatosis. These neuromas frequently are
    bilateral and occur in younger individuals than in
    spontaneous cases of acoustic neuromas.

PITFALLS:

1. During surgery for acoustic neuromas, air embolism
    can be a frustrating and dangerous problem. This
    complication is only encountered when the sitting
    position is utilized. Air emboli can be avoided by
    using the lateral park-bench position with the
    ipsilateral side up and the head turned 45° to the

contralateral side. Another alternative position is the supine position with the head turned 90° to the contralateral side.

2. When a total removal of tumor is the goal of surgery, the surgeon must drill off the superior face of the internal auditory canal. Acoustic tumors often have fingers that extend a variable distance into the canal, and failure to drill the canal may lead to incomplete tumor removal and recurrence.

3. Following successful tumor removal and preservation of the VIIth nerve, perioperative steroid therapy must not be discontinued too abruptly. Swelling in the VIIth nerve can lead to delayed facial paralysis occurring even several days after surgery. Steroids should therefore be continued in tapering doses for up to 3 weeks after surgery.

REFERENCES

1. House WF, Hitselberger WE: The neuro-otologist's view of the surgical management of acoustic neuromas. Clin Neurosurg 32:214-222, 1985.

2. King TT, Morrison AW: Translabyrinthine and transtentorial removal of acoustic nerve tumors. J Neurosurg 52:210-216, 1980.

3. Nehls DG, Spetzler RF, Shetter AG, Sonntag VKH: Application of new technology in the treatment of cerebellopontine angle tumors. Clin Neurosurg 32: 223-241, 1985.

4. Ojemann RG: Microsurgical suboccipital approach to cerebellopontine angle tumors. Clin Neurosurg 25: 461-479, 1978.

5. Samii M, Turel KE, Penkert G: Management of seventh and eighth nerve involvement by cerebellopontine angle tumors. Clin Neurosurg 32:242-272, 1985.

LOSS OF SENSATION IN THE LEFT LEG AND PROGRESSIVE WEAKNESS OF THE RIGHT ARM

CASE 2: A 59-year-old man presented with a history of progressive spinal cord dysfunction. Four years before admission he noted loss of pain and temperature sensation in the distal part of the left leg. About 1 year later he developed weakness of the right arm. During the following 2 years he had progressive weakness of the right arm and leg. One year before admission he noted decreased pain and temperature sensation in the left upper extremity. Admission neurological examination showed an elderly man with an intact mental status and normal cranial nerves. He had only antigravity strength in the intrinsic muscles of the right hand with noticeable wasting. He had proximal weakness of both the right upper and lower extremities but was ambulatory with a cane. Pain and temperature sensation was absent on the left side of the body with a level of C3, and he had a generalized diminution of position and vibratory sensation in all four extremities, more pronounced on the right side. Reflexes were hyperactive.

Neuroradiological studies demonstrated an intramedullary mass lesion in the region of the caudal medulla extending down to the level of C3 with an associated cyst.

Neuroanatomical Clue:

Knowledge of the detailed anatomy of the spinal cord allows the clinician to localize this lesion from clues offered in the history and physical examination (see diagram on next page).

6

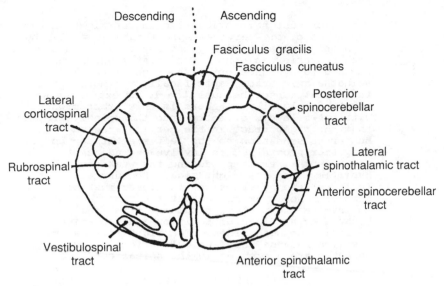

Descending : Ascending

Fasciculus gracilis
Fasciculus cuneatus

Lateral
corticospinal
tract

Posterior
spinocerebellar
tract

Rubrospinal
tract

Lateral
spinothalamic tract

Anterior spinocerebellar
tract

Vestibulospinal
tract

Anterior spinothalamic
tract

Figure 2.1

QUESTIONS:

1. Describe how the history and physical examination localize this tumor within the neuraxis. What is the approximate site of origin of this tumor?

2. The most likely diagnosis in this case is an intramedullary spinal cord tumor. What are the different types of tumors that occur in this location, and with what frequency?

3. What neuroradiological studies would be helpful in establishing this diagnosis, and what are the supporting characteristics of each study?

4. What is the surgical approach to this lesion?

5. What role does radiation treatment have in this disease?

ANSWERS:

1. The tumor must have originated in the right lateral
    funiculus of the cervical spinal cord above C5, but
    then enlarged posteriorly and medially to involve
    both posterior columns. The first symptom was
    related to dysfunction of the right lateral
    spinothalamic tract, specifically the more lateral
    the dorsal aspect because the lower extremity was
    involved primarily. Fibers in this tract cross
    within two levels of entry into the spinal cord, so
    that the right tract in the cervical region
    subserves sensation to the left side of the body.
    The tumor progressed to involve the adjacent
    corticospinal tract producing the weakness and
    hyperflexia on the right side. Because all of the
    reflexes were hyperactive, the tumor must be higher
    than C5. The exam shows that the tumor has grown
    to involve the posterior columns bilaterally
    because he had loss of position and vibration
    sensation on both sides. The right side was more
    involved because the fasciculi gracilis and
    cuneatus are uncrossed in the spinal cord.

2. About 56% of intramedullary spinal cord tumors are
    ependymomas, 27% are astrocytomas, 3% are
    hemangioblastomas, 3% are oligodendrogliomas, 2%
    are lipomas, and about 1% is of each of the
    following: metastatic tumor, dermoid tumor,
    teratoma, epidermoid tumor, cavernous hemangioma,
    and malignant glioma.

3. Fifty percent of cases will have changes on the
    routine x-rays of the spine. These include
    widening of the interpedicular distance and
    scalloping of the posterior margin of the vertebral
    bodies. The myelogram is the most useful test to
    define anintramedullary tumor. The dye column is
    narrowed symmetrically on all sides of the spinal
    cord, indicating widening of the cord diameter. If
    necessary because of complete block, the dye should
    be placed above the lesion as well as below in
    order to define the entire extent of the tumor.
    The use of metrizamide computed tomography (CT)
    will often give excellent detail as to the exact
    location of the tumor within the spinal cord rather
    than compressing it anteriorly, and CT may

demonstrate the consistency of the intramedullary
process showing a cystic rather than a solid tumor.
Spinal angiography has been of little value for
these lesions. In the future, _sagittal
reconstructions from magnetic resonance imaging
techniques may provide the most reliable and
accurate form of diagnostic tests for
intramedullary tumors_.

4. _The goal of surgical treatment is total removal of
    these tumors_. Analysis of the radiological studies
    will usually reveal the extent of the lesion.
    Surgery is then performed in the prone position
    with a generous laminectomy encompassing the entire
    area of widening on the myelogram. In most
    instances a midline myelotomy will be necessary to
    expose the tumor. Many tumors will have a clear
    plane of cleavage between spinal cord tissue and
    with carefulmicroscopic technique, the entire tumor
    can be removed. In the case of the astrocytoma, a
    plane may be found aroung the majority of the
    tumor; but in some places the tumor may blend with
    the surrounding spinal cord, and complete removal
    may not be possible.

5. Although there is some debate on this issue, _there
    is no clear indication that radiation treatment has
    any effect on benign intramedullary spinal cord
    tumors_. In fact, gliosis of the spinal cord may be
    a deleterious effect of radiation, and radiotherapy
    to the growing spine may result in severe spinal
    deformities in children. There, in the vast
    majority of cases, radiotherapy for spinal cord
    tumors is contraindicated. In the cases of
    malignant gliomas of the spinal cord, radiation
    therapy should be given, but the results in this
    disease process are uniformly poor regardless of
    the form of treatment.

PEARLS:

1. Of all intradural spinal tumors, intramedullary
    tumors represent only about 25%. Meningiomas and
    neurofibromas account for over 50%.

2. The vascular supply to the spinal cord is important
    to understand in planning any spinal surgery.
    There are 3 separate vascular territories in the
    spinal cord. The superior segment includes the
    cervical cord and first 2 thoracic segments. It is
    irrigated by the anterior spinal artery that arises
    from the intracranial vertebral arteries, a direct
    branch from the vertebral artery as it courses in
    the intertranverse foramina, and by a branch of the
    costocervical trunk. The midthoracic portion of
    the cord down to T8 is supplied primarily via a
    radicular artery located at approximately T7. The
    lower thoracolumbar area is supplied by a single
    large radicular artery (the artery of Adamkiewicz)
    that usually enters at T9 to T12.

3. The intramedullary cord tumors tend to be located
    toward the dorsal aspect of the cord. It would
    appear that the fibrous nature of the central canal
    near the ventral median raphe prevents the tumor
    from growing predominantly in this direction.
    Therefore, the growth of these tumors is toward the
    dorsal aspect of the cord, usually within
    millimeters of the pial surface. For these reasons
    intramedullary tumors can usually be easily
    accessed through a midline myelotomy.

4. The clinical syndrome produced by these tumors
    varies with the age of the patient. In children,
    the presentation is primarily one of gait
    disturbance and spinal deformity (scoliosis). Pain
    is not a prominent early feature in children. In
    adults, on the other hand, radicular pain is a
    common early symptom, followed by the insidious
    progression of increasing spinal cord dysfunction.
    Weakness and defective posterior column function
    begin early, and loss of pain and temperature
    sensation is a late finding.

PITFALLS:

1. When extensive laminectomies have been performed for the removal of spinal cord tumors, the patients should be closely followed for several years to watch for the possible development of spinal deformities. Swann-neck deformities in the cervical cases, scoliosis with the thoracic cases, and spondylolisthesis with lumbar operations have all been encountered and will usually require bracing or orthopedic intervention. Bone removal at the time of surgery as well as muscle weakness and denervation produced by the tumor contribute to deformities.

2. Even when patients with spinal cord tumors present with severe spinal cord dysfunction, operative decompression should be undertaken. Slowly growing tumors may not produce irreversible damage, and the patient may improve after tumor removal. If the tumor cannot be removed, laminectomy and duraplasty can allow for considerable cord decompression and afford some relief of symptoms.

REFERENCES

1. Connolly ES: Spinal cord tumors in adults in Youmans JR, ed.: Neurological Surgery, W.B. Saunders Co., Philadelphia, 1982, pp 3196-3214.

2. De Sousa AL, Kalsbeck JE, Mealey J, Campell RL, Hockey A: Interspinal tumors in children: a review of 81 cases. J Neurosurg 51:437-445, 1979.

3. Guidetti B, Mercuri S, Vagnozzi R: Long-term results of the surgical treatment of 129 intramedullary spinal gliomas. J Neurosurg 54:323-330, 1981.

4. Malis LI: Intramedullary spinal cord tumors. Clin Neurosurg 25:512-540, 1978.

5. Reimer R, Onofrio B: Astrocytomas of the spinal cord in children and adolescents. J Neurosurg 63:669-675, 1985.

HEADACHE AND STIFF NECK OF SUDDEN ONSET

CASE 3:   A 48-year-old woman was in excellent general
health until one evening when she experienced a sudden
severe left temporal headache accompanied by nausea and
vomiting.   Twelve hours later she presented to the
emergency room for evaluation.   She continued to
complain of mild temporal headache and neck stiffness,
but otherwise had no complaints.   The patient was alert
with normal mentation, and the remainder of the
neurological examination was entirely normal.

A computed tomography (CT) scan was performed that
showed no abnormalities.   A lumbar puncture
demonstrated grossly bloody cerebrospinal fluid (CSF).
Emergency angiography revealed a 2 cm aneurysm of the
left internal carotid artery at the level of the
posterior communicating artery.   There was no spasm,
and the aneurysm had a well-defined neck.   The
angiogram was completed within 6 hours of the patient's
arrival at the hospital.

Clue: Lateral left internal carotid angiogram:

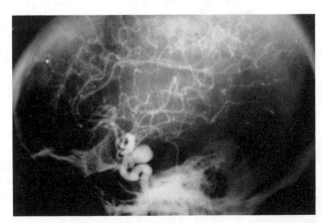

Figure 3.1

12

QUESTIONS:

1. What is the diagnosis and what is the grade of this
   patient?

2. If no treatment is offered to this patient, what are
   the primary risks that this patient will face over
   the next 2 weeks?   When is the patient most
   susceptible to each risk that you name?

3. Does the negative CT scan affect the prognosis?

4. What treatment options can be offered to this
   patient, and what are the pros and cons of each
   option?

ANSWERS:

1. <u>Subarachnoid hemorrhage (SAH) from a ruptured left posterior communicating artery aneurysm.</u> The patient is Grade I, according to the Hunt and Hess criteria:

Grade I	-	Asymptomatic, or minimal headache and slight nuchal rigidity
Grade II	-	Moderate to severe headache, nuchal rigidity, no neurological deficit other than cranial nerve palsy
Grade III	-	Drowsiness, confusion, or mild focal deficit
Grade IV	-	Stupor, moderate to severe hemiparesis, possibly early decerebrate rigidity, and vegetative disturbances
Grade V	-	Moribund appearance

2. <u>Rebleeding from the aneurysm</u> is the most immediately life threatening risk that this patient faces. The mortality from rebleeding is at least 50%. The most modern statistics demonstrate that the patient is most likely to rebleed during the first 24 hours after the initial hemorrhage, and the risk slowly diminishes over the next 14 days. During this period of time, 20-30 % of patients will have rebled. Patients who survive for 1 month after hemorrhage have approximately a 2-3% chance of rebleeding each year for the rest of their lives.

   <u>Vasospasm</u> of the major cerebral arteries is the other important risk faced by someone with SAH. Vasospasm leads to focal ischemia of the brain. Although symptomatic vasospasm is sometimes reversible, at least 50% die or are left with a major cerebral infarction. Vasospasm never presents before the 4th day after hemorrhage, has a peak incidence between 7 and 14 days after bleed, but occasionally is encountered up to 21 days after SAH.

3. In several clinical studies, when no blood is
    visualized on the initial CT scan, severe vasospasm
    was almost never encountered. In the presence of
    thick subarachnoid blood clots as seen on the CT
    scan, severe spasm is very common. Therefore this
    patient must be considered to have a reduced risk
    of developing cerebral vasospasm.

4. In the premicroscope era, cervical carotid artery
    ligation was an acceptable form of treatment for
    these types of aneurysms. However, with modern
    techniques, this form of therapy is no longer
    tenable. There are two currently acceptable
    approaches to treating this patient: (1)
    immediate craniotomy and clip ligation of the
    aneurysm, or (2) conservative treatment for 10-14
    days prior to craniotomy for clipping of the
    aneurysm.

    Early surgery has the advantage of preventing
the risk of rebleeding from the aneurysm and
thereby eliminates a major cause of morbidity and
mortality in this group of patients. However,
early surgery has not been shown to affect the
incidence of delayed cerebral ischemia from
vasospasm. The major drawback of early aneurysm
surgery is that the operation is technically more
difficult than delayed surgery. The brain is more
tense, more difficult to retract, and therefore
more easily injured.

    Delayed surgery can be performed with a very low
morbidity, because all candidates for this type of
treatment will have passed the critical period for
cerebral vasospasm, and the operation is
technically easier than with early surgery.
However, the patients continue to be at risk for
rebleeding from the aneurysm while awaiting
surgery.

    Currently it seems that the overall management
morbidity-mortality for these two approaches to the
aneurysm patient is about the same. Further
studies will be needed to clarify which approach if
any is superior.

PEARLS:

1. Antifibrinolytic agents have been advocated for the
    prevention of rebleeding from recently ruptured
    aneurysms. Most of the data that have been
    accumulated about these agents demonstrate that
    although they might reduce rebleeding (this fact
    has not been clearly established), they definitely
    increase the incidence of ischemic complications
    after SAH. Overall antifibrinolytic agents have
    failed to demonstrate any effectiveness in reducing
    the morbidity of aneurysmal SAH.

2. Calcium channel blockers have been used to prevent
    cerebral vasospasm after SAH. One multicenter
    clinical trial showed effectiveness of this agent
    in preventing cerebral ischemia after SAH, even
    though angiographic vasospasm was not reduced.
    However, numerous laboratory studies have failed to
    show that calcium channel blockers can prevent or
    reverse experimental vasospasm, and newer clinical
    trials of early surgery and nimodipine treatment
    have demonstrated that there is no reduction in the
    incidence of ischemic complications experienced by
    treated patients. Presently, the effectiveness of
    these agents cannot be supported.

3. Volume expansion for the symptomatic treatment of
    patients with delayed ischemic deficits after SAH
    has shown some merit. Several studies have
    demonstrated that after SAH patients with delayed
    ischemia tend to have reduced circulating blood
    volume. It seems logical that expansion of the
    blood volume would improve cardiac circulation
    through a vasospastic vascular bed that is devoid
    of normal autoregulation. Indeed clinical studies
    have demonstrated the effectiveness of this form of
    therapy.

    In most patients a central venous catheter is
    all that is required, although Swan-Ganz monitoring
    may be necessary in patients with marginal cardiac
    reserve. The hematocrit is generally maintained in
    the low 30s and central venous pressure is elevated
    to around 12 mm H_2O with crystalloid, colloid, or

blood products depending on the clinical situation. If the patient has a previously clipped aneurysm, hypertension can be induced with dopamine or similar agents if volume expansion alone does not produce clinical improvement.

PITFALLS:

1. Even when the patient does well after SAH and has successful clipping of the aneurysm, she may deteriorate weeks or months later. Often these patients develop confusion, lethargy, or loss of ambition. In this situation delayed hydrocephalus is often responsible. Hydrocephalus is secondary to the blood in the subarachnoid space, which interferes with absorption of CSF by the arachnoid granulations.

2. Postoperative angiography is critical in cases of giant aneurysms, especially when only the neck if visualized at surgery and the fundus of the aneurysm has not been excised. Failure to perform this study leaves the patient at risk because the aneurysm may be incompletely clipped, a major vessel may be compromised, or the patient may have severe asymptomatic spasm.

REFERENCES

1. Allen GS, Ahn HS, Preziosi TJ, et al.: Cerebral arterial spasm - a controlled trial of nimodipine in patients with subarachnoid hemorrhage. N Engl J Med 308:619-624, 1983.

2. Drake CG: Management of cerebral aneurysm. Stroke 1:273-283, 1981.

3. Fisher CM, Roberson GH, Ojemann RG: Relation of cerebral vasospasm to subarachnoid hemorrhage visualized by computerized tomographic scanning. Neurosurgery 6:1-9, 1980.

4. Hunt WE, Hess RM: Surgical risk as related to time
   of intervention in the repair of intracranial
   aneurysms. J Neurosurg 28:14-20, 1968.

5. Kassell NJ, Peerless SJ, Durward QJ, et al.:
   Treatment of ischemic deficits from vasospasm with
   intravascular volume expansion and induced arterial
   hypertension. Neurosurgery 11:337-341, 1982.

6. Kassell NJ, Torner JC, Adams HP, et al.:
   Antifibrinolytic therapy in the acute phase
   following aneurysmal subarachnoid hemorrhage:
   preliminary observations from the Cooperative
   Aneurysm Study. J Neurosurg 61:225-230, 1984.

7. Ljunggren B, Brandt L, Kagstrom E, Sundbarg G:
   Results of early operations for ruptured aneurysms.
   J Neurosurg 54:473-479, 1981.

8. Solomon RA, Fink ME: Current strategies for the
   management of aneurysmal subarachnoid hemorrhage.
   Arch Neurol 44:769-774, 1987.

DEMENTIA, GAIT DISTURBANCE, AND INCONTINENCE OF URINE

CASE 4: A 70-year-old woman presented with a history of memory impairment and difficulty walking. Several months before admission the patient's family noted that she had become forgetful and confused. About this time, the patient began to have difficulties walking and had fallen several times. Finally, 1 week before admission she had become incontinent of urine. There was no history of head trauma or other neurological problems. She had noted no visual changes or headaches.

Examination revealed a pleasant, elderly woman. She was alert and oriented, but had marked difficulty with serial 7s and was unable to concentrate on more complex questions. There was no papilledema and the fundi were normal. The rest of the cranial nerve exam was unremarkable. Motor strength and tone were normal. There were no sensory deficits. The tendon reflexes were brisk and plantor reflexes were extensor. Romberg's sign was absent. The patient was able to stand without assistance but walked with small, staggering steps and fell repeatedly to both sides on tandem gait.

A computed tomography (CT) scan revealed dilation of the lateral and fourth ventricles. No cortical atrophy was present. On lumbar puncture, the opening pressure was 140 mm. Examination of the cerebrospinal fluid (CSF) was unremarkable. Following removal of 50 ml of fluid, the patient showed improvement in both tandem gait and mental status examinations.

QUESTIONS:

1. What is the most likely diagnosis in this patient? What are the various causes of this condition?

2. What is the pathogenesis of this condition? How can the apparent paradox of ventriculomegaly in the setting of normal CSF pressure be explained?

3. What is the treatment of this condition? Which patients will most likely benefit from therapy?

4. What are the complications of treatment?

ANSWERS:

1. The triad of dementia, gait disturbance, and
    urinary incontinence in the setting of
    hydrocephalus with normal CSF pressure--or normal
    pressure hydrocephalus (NPH)--was characterized by
    Adams and coworkers in 1965. NPH may follow
    subarachnoid hemorrhage or head trauma but in at
    least one third of cases is believed to be caused
    by a fibrosing arachnoiditis of unknown etiology.
    Rarer causes include prior surgery, meningitis,
    aqueductal stenosis, or Arnold-Chiari
    malformations.

    NPH may develop at any time following one of its
    known causes, occasionally presenting years after
    the precipitating event. The mean age of onset of
    idiopathic NPH is 68 years; no sex differences are
    seen. The mental status changes range from minimal
    impairment in concentration of insidious onset to
    frank obtundation or coma. The dementia is usually
    progressive, however, and the patients may become
    apathetic or lethargic. Patients typically have a
    wide-based gait, take short steps and are unable to
    perform tandem walking. Urinary incontinence,and
    occasionally fecal incontinence, tend to develop
    later in the course of the disease. Both brisk
    tendon reflexes and extensor plantar responses may
    be seen.

2. The exact pathogenesis of NPH is unknown. However,
    the basic defect appears to be an incomplete
    obstruction of CSF flow within the ventricular
    system or at the base of the brain, with a
    resulting pressure gradient between the ventricular
    and subdural spaces. There is no appreciable
    defect in CSF absorption.

    The normal CSF pressure may reflect a
    compensatory mechanism in which CSF formation has
    equilibrated with absorption, allowing the once
    elevated CSF pressure to return to normal.
    However, the force exerted by the ventricles on the
    surrounding parenchyma--given by the Laplace
    equation as ventricular area multiplied by CSF

pressure--remains elevated as a result of the expanded size of the ventricles. This increased force may contribute to the clinical abnormalities seen in NPH.

Although CSF pressure at the time of a single lumbar puncture may be normal, continuous monitoring has demonstrated that patients with NPH can develop transient increases in intracranial pressure (ICP). The contribution of these waves of increased pressure to the development or maintenance of the hydrocephalus in NPH is not clear.

3. Ventricular shunting has been used with variable success in patients with NPH. Ventriculoperitoneal shunting is the preferred method in most patients with NPH, although ventriculoatrial shunting may also be used. After placement in the ventricle, the shunt is tunneled subcutaneously to the abdomen where the end is inserted into the peritoneal cavity. The draining fluid is absorbed over the surface of the peritoneum. A one-way, pressure dependent valve is placed in the shunt to ensure unidirectional flow.

Patients with an identifiable cause of NPH, in particular, subarachnoid hemorrhage, usually improve with shunting. Numerous tests or historical criteria have been used to select those patients with idiopathic NPH who will benefit from shunting. Patients who present primarily with a gait disturbance and who have little or no dementia or incontinence are good candidates for shunting. Improvement in gait abnormalities or mental status following a single or serial lumbar tap tests (in which 50 ml of CSF are removed) is also predictive of a good result. Infusion manometry, radionuclide cisternography, and measurement of cerebral blood flow also have been utilized.

Overall, 65% of patients with NPH from an identifiable cause improve with shunting, whereas only 41% benefit when the cause is unknown.

4. Up to 44% of shunted patients will develop
    complications. These include infection, shunt
    malfunction, subdural hematoma or hygroma, and
    seizures. Shunt patients who detiorate clinically
    should have a CT scan to rule out a hematoma or
    hygroma that might require surgical drainage. In
    addition, a lumbar puncture to measure pressure and
    to look for evidence of meningitis may be
    indicated. A "shunt series," or serial plain films
    along the course of the shunt, can identify
    disruptions or kinks in the tubing.

PEARLS:

1. Headache and papilledema are typically not seen in
    patients with NPH and their presence should raise
    suspicion of another diagnosis. Localizing
    neurological signs also suggest another diagnosis
    as most patients with NPH have a nonfocal
    examination.

2. Many patients benefit from shunting despite no
    postoperative reduction in ventricular size,
    improvement resulting from an decrease in pressure
    alone.

PITFALLS:

1. Hydrocephalus as well as dementia, incontinence,
    and gait abnormalities may all occur with
    Alzheimer's disease. As a result, it is often
    difficult to distinguish NPH from Alzheimer's
    disease. This is essential because shunt placement
    is not indicated for patients with Alzheimer's
    disease. Sulcal atrophy with little
    ventriuculomegaly on CT scan, accompanied by
    minimal gait abnormalities on exam, suggest
    Alzheimer's disease.

2. Failure to improve following shunting in patients
    with NPH may be the result of a coexistent
    degenerative brain disease, in particular
    Alzheimer's disease. Failure may also result if
    treatment is not initiated soon enough.

3. Sudden reduction of ventricular pressure after
    shunt placement may cause rupture of dural veins
    with subsequent subdural hematoma. For this
    reason, patients are kept in a horizontal position
    after shunt placement for up to a day, followed by
    gradual head elevation.

REFERENCES

1. Adams RD, Fisher CM, Hakim S, Ojemann RG, and Sweet
    WH: Symptomatic occult hydrocephalus with "normal"
    cerebrospinal fluid pressure. N Engl J Med 273:117-
    126, 1965.

2. Adams RD, Victor M. Principles of neurology
    (3rd ed). McGraw-Hill, New York; 1985. pp.466-
    467.

3. Hakim S, Adams RD. The special clinical problem of
    symptomatic hydrocephalus with normal
    cerebrospinal fluid pressure. Observation on
    cerebrospinal fluid hydrodynamics. J Neurol Sci
    2:307-327, 1965.

4. Huckman MS. Normal pressure hydrocephalus:
    evaluation of diagnostic and prognostic tests. Am
    J Neuroradiol 2:385-395, 1981.

5. Long DM. Aging in the nervous system. Neurosurgery
    17:348-354, 1985.

6. Ojemann RG, and Black PM. Evaluation of patient
    with dementia and treatment of normal pressure
    hydrocephalus. In Neurosurgery. Wilkins RH,
    Rengachary SS, eds. McGraw-Hill, New York, 1985.
    pp.316-321.

7. Wikkelso C, Andersson H, Blomstrand C, et al: Normal
    pressure hydrocephalus: predictive value of the
    cerebrospinal fluid tap-test. Acta Neurolog
    Scand 73:566-573, 1986.

INTRACTABLE TEMPORAL LOBE EPILEPSY

CASE 5: A 25-year-old woman presented with a history of seizures. Three years before admission she had a brief generalized tonic-clonic ("grand mal") seizure. Subsequently she began having weekly episodes which lasted 2-20 minutes, characterized by awareness of a "strange smell" followed by nausea and a poorly described "strange feeling." She did not lose consciousness. Additional history included frequent (several times per week) attacks of unprovoked anger or rage lasting minutes to hours. Past medical history was otherwise unremarkable including details of gestation, birth, and postnatal development.

Neurological examination was normal. In particular the patient had normal speech and memory and full visual fields.

Clue:

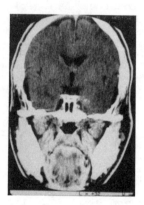

Figure 5.1

QUESTIONS:

1. What type(s) of seizures does this patient have?

2. What diagnostic tests would be indicated in the initial evaluation (see Clue)?

ADDITIONAL CASE HISTORY: A computed tomography (CT)
scan shortly after the single generalized seizure
revealed a 2 cm calcified mass in the mesial aspect of
the right anterior temporal lobe.   An interictal
electroencephalogram (EEG) revealed focal spikes and
sharp waves from the right anterior temporal region.
Over the 3 years prior to her current evaluation, the
patient was treated with various anticonvulsant drugs,
singly and in combination, including phenytoin,
carbamazepine, and phenobarbital.   There was no
definite effect on seizure frequency or pattern.   A
repeat CT scan revealed no interim change in the right
temporal lobe calcified mass.

QUESTIONS:

3. What is the most likely pathological diagnosis of
   the lesion?

4. What (if any) surgical therapy is indicated for this
   patient?

5. What further test(s) should be done prior to
   surgery?

ANSWERS:

1. This patient's initial seizure was a generalized
    tonic-clonic attack. However, the remainder of her
    seizures would be categorized as <u>partial seizures</u>.
    Because she apparently did not lose consciousness,
    they would be further classified as "simple"
    partial seizures, although more detailed
    information might indicate that level of awareness
    was altered, in which case the seizures would be
    categorized as "complex" partial.

    Thus, the first seizure, although generalized,
    was most likely secondary spread from the right
    temporal focus. Use of anticonvulsant drugs,
    although ineffective against the partial attacks,
    probably suppressed further generalization. Simple
    or complex partial seizures of temporal lobe origin
    have a wide variety of manifestations. They
    generally have two unique features that allow them
    to be differentiated from other seizure types.
    First, they are usually initiated by a transient
    subjective experience (an illusion, hallucination,
    dyscognitive state such as déjà vu or affective
    experience such as fear or anxiety). Less often, a
    brief motor phenomenon may occur (e.g., facial
    twitch). Such symptoms are really simple partial
    seizures, but when they occur as a prelude to
    further symptoms and behaviors, they are commonly
    referred to as an "aura." The second feature
    represents a period of confused behavior during
    which the person is unresponsive to the environment
    and typically carries out complex but purposeless
    automatic type movements which may include walking,
    chewing, swallowing, or vocalization and for which
    there is amnesia. The aura is often a clue to the
    anatomical location of the seizure focus. For
    example an unusual smell (as with this patient) is
    characteristic of a discharge originating in the
    uncus or hippocampus (so-called "uncinate
    seizures"). This patient's rage attacks are
    unlikely to be seizures but rather episodes of
    behavioral dyscontrol due to temporal lobe
    pathology. Study of a large series of patients

with epilepsy found only a 2.4% incidence of rage or aggression episodes, and these were typically not ictal.

2. The evaluation of this patient should include a CT scan of the brain with and without contrast and an EEG. CT scans in patients with complex partial seizures of temporal lobe origin demonstrate an abnormality in 63% of cases. Abnormal findings include focal atrophy, calcification, malformations, hydrocephalus, tumors, and vascular anomalies. The application of magnetic resonance imaging (MRI) may increase the sensitivity for certain types of lesions, especially atrophic or gliotic ones, not well visualized by CT. Thus an MRI scan should be obtained in patients with focal seizures who have a negative CT or alternatively may be employed as an initial test of choice.

EEGs in patients with epilepsy are abnormal in 55% of patients awake and in 75% when asleep. The yield is increased with longer recordings such as telemetry monitoring, and sometimes by tapering anticonvulsant medications. When a temporal lobe focus is suspected, nasopharyngeal (or sphenoidal) electrodes may be used to detect abnormalities arising from the medial temporal lobe. Thus, the EEG should include a sleep recording and use of anterior temporal leads.

3. The majority of patients with partial seizures and a unilateral temporal lobe EEG focus have mesial temporal (or incisural) sclerosis. Histologically this is an area of neuronal loss and gliosis involving uncus, amygdala, and hippocampus. The pathophysiology of this finding is not certain. Other pathologic entities encountered include occult tumors, hamartomas, polymicrogyria, acquired scars, and arteriovenous malformations. This patient's seizures, temporal EEG focus, and mass on CT suggest a hamartoma or possibly low grade tumor (e.g., Grade I astrocytoma).

4. Seizures persist greater than 2 years despite institution of vigorous anticonvulsant regimens (including combination therapy) in approximately 33% of patients with epilepsy. Frequently

recurring seizures can cause neuronal damage or
lead to status epilepticus, which carries with it
a 10% mortality risk and, if prolonged, serious
neurological sequelae.

Furthermore, uncontrolled seizures impose
incalculable psychosocial limitations on the
patients.

Surgical therapy should be considered in any
patient with focal epilepsy whose seizures remain
disabling despite optimal medical treatment for 2
years. Surgery may be considered earlier when
imaging studies demonstrate significant pathology
since in such cases successful medical management
is unlikely. Furthermore, increased awareness of
the diverse nature of such lesions probably
warrants biopsy for definitive diagnosis.

Cortical resection of epileptogenic foci
represents by far the most effective treatment for
uncontrolled epilepsy. Indications include a
seizure focus that is located in an area amenable
to resection without deficit and sufficiently
circumscribed that total removal is likely. In
temporal lobe cases, the contralateral homologous
area must be intact. Patients with complex partial
seizures and a unilateral temporal lobe EEG focus
constitute 80% of all cortical resections.
Patients who fail to demonstrate a well localized
EEG focus, have bilateral foci, or have a focus
that is not consistent with CT scan findings or
clinical diagnosis should be considered for
transient or prolonged direct brain recordings
(DBRs) using subdural or depth electrodes. In one
series of patients with bitemporal EEG foci, DBR
identified 88% of all major seizures as arising
from one side. The standard technique for temporal
lobectomy involves en bloc resection of the
anterior (up to 5.5 cm on the dominant side and 6.0
cm on the nondominant side) and medial (including
uncus, hippocampus, and amygdala) temporal lobe,
often sparing the superior temporal gyrus. After
temporal lobectomy, over 75% of patients experience
major improvement and most are seizure free. The

complication rate of temporal lobectomy is low,
with reports of a 0.2% mortality and anywhere from
1-16% morbidity (infection or some degree of
neurological deficit such as hemiparesis, aphasia,
or memory impairment). In appropriately selected
patients, potential benefits of this operation
clearly outweigh the risks.

5. Most surgeons believe that the "Wada test" should
    be carried out prior to temporal lobectomy. This
    test involves sequential injection of amobarbital
    into each carotid artery using the technique for
    cerebral angiography. The purpose of this test is
    to identify the hemisphere of speech dominance and
    to determine whether the temporal lobe to be
    operated on is required for memory function. This
    knowledge may not prevent operation, but it will
    indicate the necessity for careful functional
    mapping at the time of cortical resection.

ADDITIONAL CASE HISTORY: A Wada test prior to
operation in this woman revealed left hemisphere
dominance for speech and that the left hemisphere alone
was able to support memory function. A right temporal
craniotomy was carried out under general anesthesia
with resection of the anterior 5 cm of the temporal
lobe, including the medial components (e.g., uncus,
anterior hippocampus, and amygdala) and excluding the
superior temporal gyrus. Following resection,
electrocorticography detected no epileptogenic
activity. The patient did well postoperatively and has
been seizure free for over 1 year. Cautious taper of
anticonvulsant drugs is now planned. The pathological
diagnoses included mesial temporal sclerosis, a
hamartomatous lesion, and small area consistent with a
Grade I astrocytoma.

PEARLS:

1. Differentiate partial (focal) from generalized onset seizures.

2. Select appropriate anticonvulsant drug according to seizure type: carbamazepine or phenytoin for focal seizures and valproate for generalized seizures.

3. Increase anticonvulsant drugs according to clinical progress as determined by seizure frequency and evidence of toxicity.

4. Seek focal anatomical abnormalities with CT or MRI and localized functional abnormalities using EEG.

5. Consider cortical resection in patients with disabling refractory focal seizures.

PITFALLS:

1. Failure to design rational treatment protocols and goals.

2. Failure to obtain adequate imaging studies to detect focal pathology in patients with longstanding seizures.

REFERENCES

1. Adams RD, Victor M.: Principles of Neurology. New York, McGraw-Hill, pp 233-254, 1985.
2. Annegers JF, Hauser WA, Elveback LT, Kurland LT. Remission and relapse of seizures in epilepsy. In Wada JA Penry JK eds Advances in Epileptology X. New York, 1980 Raven Press pp.143-147.
3. Goldring S: Epilepsy surgery. Clin. Neurosurg 31:369-88, 1984.
4. Ojemann GA: Surgical treatment of epilepsy, In Wilkins RH, Rengachary SS, eds. Neurosurgery. New York, McGraw-Hill pp 2517-2527, 1985.

5. Okuma T, and Kumashiro H: Natural history
   and prognosis of epilepsy. In Wada JA,
   Penry JK, <u>Advances in Epileptology X</u>. New York, Raven
   Press, pp 135-141, 1980.

PROPTOSIS, DECREASED VISUAL ACUITY, AND CAFÉ AU LAIT SPOTS

CASE 6: An 8-year-old boy presented with proptosis (exophthalmos) of his right eye. His mother first noted a definite proptosis 2 weeks before admission but felt that his eye had looked abnormal for several months. There was no history of double vision, pain in the eye, headache, nausea, or vomiting.

On examination, the boy had a painless, non-pulsatile proptosis of the right eye. No chemosis, vascular injection, or bruits were appreciated. Fundoscopic examination showed disc pallor on the right with no evidence of papilledema. Visual acuity was 20/20 on the left and 20/200 on the right. Visual fields were intact to confrontation. Examination of the pupils and extraocular muscles was normal. The rest of the cranial nerve examination was unremarkable, as were the motor and sensory examinations. On general physical examination, several café au lait colored macules were noted over the trunk.

Plain radiographs of the orbit showed enlargement of the right optic foramen. Computed tomography revealed that the right optic nerve was widened and nodular in appearance from the globe to the apex of the orbit. The sella turcica and optic chiasm were normal.

NEUROANATOMICAL CLUE:

The absence of bitemporal hemianopia on physical examination suggests sparing of the optic chiasm.

QUESTIONS:

1. What is the differential diagnosis of proptosis?
   How would pain, pulsation, or vascular injection in
   the eye alter your differential?
   What is the likely diagnosis in this child given the
   finding of café au lait spots on examination?

2. What is the natural history of this child's
   condition?
   What are the clinical and radiographic hallmarks of
   this condition?
   What is the surgical management of this disease?

3. How would involvement of the optic chiasm alter your
   therapy?

4. Discuss the role of radiotherapy in this condition.

ANSWERS:

1. Proptosis may be caused by an orbital neoplasm, cellulitis, mucocoele (from sinus obstruction), cavernous sinus thrombosis, histiocytosis, caroticocavernous fistula, arteriovenous malformation, thyrotoxicosis, or myxedema.

    Meningiomas (40%), hemangiomas (10%), and gliomas (5%) are the most common primary tumors of the orbit; neurofibromas, epidermoids, lipomas, and primary carcinomas occur less frequently. Metastatic lesions from lung, breast, pancreas, melanoma, and (in children) neuroblastoma may also be seen.

    Orbital pain is rarely found with a primary orbital tumor. Its presence should raise suspicion of an invasive carcinoma or, if accompanied by redness of the eye, orbital pseudotumor. This condition is characterized by a nonspecific chronic inflammation in the orbit of unknown etiology that usually responds to steroid therapy.

    Orbital pulsations and vascular injection or chemosis suggest an orbital arteriovenous malformation or caroticocavernous fistula. A caroticocavernous fistula may occur following basal skull fracture or spontaneous rupture of the intracavernous carotid artery in elderly hypertensives.

    The presence of café au lait spots in this child suggests the diagnosis of neurofibromatosis. In this setting, the most likely etiology of the proptosis is optic nerve glioma.

2. Optic nerve gliomas represent 5% of all pediatric intracranial tumors, occur predominantly in the first and second decades of life, and are associated with neurofibromatosis. The natural history of optic nerve gliomas is variable, although they usually are slow growing and may demonstrate long-term stabilization and even spontaneous regression in some cases.

Patients commonly present with the gradual onset of proptosis and decreasing visual acuity. Examination usually reveals disc pallor; nerve palsies and papilledema are rare. Enlargement of the optic canal may be seen on plain radiographs. Thickening of the entire optic nerve, fusiform dilation of the nerve, or nodularity is visible on computed tomography. In addition, computed tomography may detect contralateral lesions that are clinically silent, or document chiasmal involvement or obstructive hydrocephalus in more extensive cases.

Although radiotherapy alone has been advocated for the treatment of unilateral gliomas restricted to the optic nerve, transcranial resection with preservation of the globe and chiasm is generally perceived to be the treatment of choice in the face of progressive proptosis and visual loss.

3. Approximately two-thirds of optic nerve gliomas will have some degree of chiasmal involvement on presentation. These patients may develop bitemporal field deficits, obstructive hydrocephalus, as well as endocrine deficits secondary to hypothalamic involvement. Computed tomography will often show chiasmal enlargement but may miss smaller, non-enhancing lesions.

Surgical intervention in cases of chiasmal involvement is indicated only for tissue diagnosis or decompression of obstructive hydrocephalus. Because of their dangerous location, these tumors carry a worse prognosis than gliomas limited to the optic nerve, although some evidence exists that they are biologically more aggressive as well.

4. Radiotherapy is the treatment of choice for optic gliomas that are bilateral or invlove the optic chiasm. Most patients will demonstrate improved or stabilized vision following treatment, and long-term remission may be expected in up to 90% of patients. Supplemental radiotherapy following excision of tumors confined to a single optic nerve has also been recommended, particularly if a tumor-free margin in the proximal specimen cannot be

obtained. The long-term side effects of radiotherapy in children are difficult to assess but may include mental retardation and endocrinological impairment.

PEARLS:

1. Hydrocephalus on presentation of an optic glioma is considered a poor prognostic sign, associated with an increased incidence of recurrence.

2. The superior ramus of the oculomotor nerve (supplying the superior rectus and levator palpebrae muscles) lies on top of the optic nerve, while the inferior ramus lies beneath it. The abducens nerve courses laterally to supply the lateral rectus muscle. This permits surgical access to the optic nerve from the medial side with sparing of the innervation of the extraocular muscles.

3. The direction of proptosis in tumors of the optic nerve is outward along the orbital axis. Displacement in the coronal plane suggests a process extrinsic to the nerve, muscle cone, or apex. For instance, a lacrimal tumor would result in inferior and medial displacement of the orbit.

4. Diplopia caused by a benign orbital tumor may reflect mechanical displacement of the globe rather than an extraocular nerve palsy.

PITFALLS:

1. As many as 20% of orbital biopsies are done for orbital pseudotumor.

2. Because of potential intracranial seeding, malignant orbital tumors (as in metastatic lesions) should not be resected via a transcranial approach.

3. Only 1% of patients with unilateral proptosis in the general population will have an optic nerve glioma. The most common cause of unilateral proptosis is thyrotoxicosis.

REFERENCES

1. Degowin EL, Degowin RL: Bedside diagnostic examination. New York, Macmillan, 1981, p 88.

2. Horwich A, Bloom HJ: Optic gliomas: radiation therapy and prognosis. Int J Radiat Oncol Biol Phys 11:1067-79, 1985.

3. Housepian EM, Trokel SL, Jakobiec FO, Hilal SK: Tumors of the orbit.   In: Youman JR, ed. Neurological Surgery. Philadelphia, Saunders, 1982, p 3024-3064.

4. Patten J. Neurological differential diagnosis. London, Harold Starke Limited, 1977, p 38.

5. Tenny RT, Laws ER, Younge BR, Rush JA: The neurosurgical management of optic glioma: results in 104 patients. J Neurosurg 57:452:458, 1982.

6. Weiss L, Sagerman RH, King GA, Chung CT, Dubowy RL: Controversy in the management of optic nerve glioma. Cancer 59:1000-1004, 1987.

SLOWLY PROGRESSIVE NUMBNESS ON RIGHT SIDE AND GAIT DIFFICULTY

CASE 7: A 53-year-old man was in excellent health until 6 months prior to admission when he noted the onset of numbness and tingling in his right foot. Over the next several months the numbness slowly progressed and extended proximally to involve the entire right side of his body to the shoulder level. Over the same period the patient experienced progressive gait difficulty. In the 3 weeks preceding admission the patient noted the onset of urinary frequency and hesitancy and had 2 episodes of urinary incontinence.

Neurological examination revealed increased tone in the left arm and in both legs. Deep tendon reflexes were abnormally brisk in both legs with extensor plantar responses bilaterally. The patient's gait was spastic with marked circumduction of the left leg. Sensory testing demonstrated diminished vibratory and light touch perception on the right up to the shoulder level.

Plain films of the cervical spine revealed moderate degenerative changes and prominent spondylitic bars at the C3-C4 and C6-C7 interspaces. Iohexal myelography demonstrated significant ventral extradural defects at the C3-C4 and C6-C7 interspaces. Computed tomography of the cervical spine showed compression of the spinal cord by both spondylitic bars.

A decompressive laminectomy was performed with removal of the C3-C7 laminae. Postoperatively, he has done well with improvement of his gait and return of normal bladder function. He still has significant spasticity and requires a cane because of continued deficits of position sense.

NEUROANATOMICAL CLUE: The normal sagittal (anteroposterior) diameter of the lower cervical canal ranges from 12 to 22 mm. The average diameter is 17 mm. The normal sagittal diameter of the spinal cord at this level is 10 mm. Narrowing of the spinal canal by herniated disc, osteophyte formation, or thickened ligamentum flavum to diameters below 11 mm. will usually produce symptomatic spinal cord compression.

QUESTIONS:

1. What is the etiology of cervical spondylosis?

2. List the classical clinical triad of cervical spondylosis.

3. What radiological tests are helpful in making the diagnosis of cervical spondylosis?

4. What is the treatment of cervical spondylosis?

ANSWERS:

1.   Cervical spondylosis is a chronic degenerative
     disorder involving the cervical spine. The common
     pathological link between the different clinical
     forms of cervical spondylosis is degeneration of
     the intervertebral disc. The disc degeneration
     leads to a progressive narrowing of the disc space
     and ultimately results in contact between adjacent
     cervical vertebrae. Reactive changes occur at these
     sites of contact in the form of bony overgrowths.
     These bony overgrowths, termed osteophytes or
     spondylitic bars, may encroach on the spinal canal
     or intervertebral foramina producing myelopathy or
     radiculopathy, respectively. Rarely, an osteophyte
     may cause intermittent symptomatic vertebral artery
     compression.

         Thus, cervical spondylosis can be considered as
     a form of osteoarthritis. These degenerative
     changes can be appreciated on radiographic and
     autopsy studies in most of the adult population
     over the age of 50 years. The severity of these
     changes tend to increase with age. Obviously, the
     majority of people over the age of 50 years do not
     exhibit symptoms of spinal cord or root
     compression. The development of symptoms depends
     not only on the severity of degenerative changes
     but also on the existing sagittal diameter of the
     spinal canal. Patients whose sagittal diameter is
     in the low normal range (under 15 mm) are more
     prone to develop symptomatic cervical spondylosis.

2.   The clinical triad of symptomatic cervical
     spondylosis includes: 1) neck pain and stiffness,
     2) arm pain, and 3) spastic lower extremity
     weakness. It is important to note that any one of
     these features may predominate the clinical picture
     in a particular patient and, in many patients, not
     all of the components of the clinical triad are
     present. It is also important to appreciate that
     there are many clinical variations within each
     symptom complex. Thus, neck pain may be described
     by the patient as a stiff neck or as simply a
     limitation of movement. The patient may even
     complain of an occipital headache. Most commonly,
     the pain is localized to the neck and is

aggravated by movement. There is frequently
radiation across the superior border of both
scapulae. Brachalgia may be in a radicular
distribution but it may also be diffuse in nature,
particularly when the C7 root is involved.
Occasionally, numbness, and not pain, may be the
only symptom of nerve root involvement. Spasticity
in the legs often develops insidiously and usually
affects both legs equally. Initially, the patient
may complain of leg cramps, fatigue, or stiffness
during exercise or prolonged walking. Only with
severe spinal cord compression will the classic
stooped posture and markedly spastic gait become
apparent. Disturbances of micturition, heralded by
urinary frequency and hesitancy and, rarely,
incontinence, are also signs of severe disease.

3. Plain films of the cervical spine are useful in the
    initial screening of patients with suspected
    cervical spondylosis. These will permit accurate
    measurement of the diameter of the cervical spinal
    canal and, because most spondylitic osteophytes
    result from bony overgrowth, the identification of
    these osteophytes will also be possible with plain
    films. Oblique projections are useful in
    identifying bony encroachment and narrowing of the
    intervertebral foramina. If spinal cord compression
    is secondary to a herniated disc or a noncalcified
    thickened annulus fibrosis, however, cervical spine
    films may be unremarkable. More recently, magnetic
    resonance imaging (MRI) has been employed in the
    initial evaluation of patients with cervical
    spondylosis. This noninvasive modality, by imaging
    both the osteophyte and the spinal cord, allow a
    quantification of the degree of spinal cord
    compression. MRI is still somewhat insensitive,
    however, in imaging root compression within the
    intervertebral foramen. Iohexal myelography is
    still the definitive radiological test in assessing
    the severity of cervical spondylosis. When combined
    with postmyelography computerized tomography, the
    surgeon is best able to determine the appropriate
    level and degree of both spinal cord and nerve root
    compression.

4. The treatment of cervical spondylosis is either conservative <u>medical management or surgical decompression</u>. Conservative management includes non-narcotic analgesics for pain control and cervical immobilization, usually with a soft collar. Physical therapy, consisting of cervical isometric exercises, aimed at strengthening the paravertebral musculature is also helpful. In general, these conservative measures benefit those patients with relatively mild spondylosis in which pain is the predominant symptom.

Surgical decompression is reserved for those patients who have failed conservative therapy or who have more severe disease with documented spinal cord or nerve root compression. Removal of the spondylitic bar may be accomplished by an anterior approach through the neck. The osteophyte is removed through the disc space. An interbody fusion with an autologous bone graft from the iliac crest may be performed. The anterior approach is appropriate for more focal disease affecting the middle cervical segments. Spondylosis involving more than 3 intervertebral segments or involving the upper or lower portions of the cervical spine is better treated with a posterior decompressive laminectomy.

PEARLS:

1. <u>The C5-C6 and the C6-C7 interspaces are the most commonly affected</u> levels in patients with cervical spondylosis. The severity of degenerative changes seen at these levels reflects the finding that the mobility of the cervical spine is greatest at these levels.

2. As is the case with other structural lesions affecting the spinal cord, early recognition and prompt treatment of cervical spondylosis offers a better chance of a good result. Appropriate surgical decompression in a patient with longstanding neurological deficit has little chance of reversing the deficit.

PITFALLS:

1. Excessive manipulation of the neck in patients with cervical spondylosis, particularly under general anesthesia, should be avoided. <u>Extension of the neck causes an inward buckling of the ligamentum flavum which further narrows the diameter of the spinal canal and may produce irreversible spinal cord damage</u> from compression.

2. Extensive laminectomies which extend laterally to involve the facet joints place the patient at risk for the development of delayed cervical instability in the form of a <u>SWAN NECK DEFORMITY</u>. All patients should undergo periodic plain film examination to identify the development of delayed cervical instability.

REFERENCES

1. Cloward RB: New method of diagnosis and treatment of cervical disc disease. Clin Neurosurg 8:93-132, 1962.

2. Fager CAL: Results of adequate posterior decompression in the relief of spondylitic cervical myelopathy. J Neurosurg 38:364-369, 1973.

3. Friedenberg Z, Miller W: Degenerative disc disease of the cervical spine. J Bone Joint Surg 45A:1171-1178, 1963.

4. Lees F, Turner J: Natural history and prognosis of cervical spondylosis. Br Med J 2:1607-1610, 1963.

5. Pallis C, Jones AM, Spillane JD: Cervical spondylosis: incidence and implications. Brain 77:274-289, 1954.

ACUTE ONSET OF MIDBACK PAIN AND HEADACHE WITH ASSOCIATED NAUSEA AND VOMITING

CASE 8: A 27-year-old previously healthy woman presented with the acute onset of severe midback pain and headache. There were associated nausea and vomiting.

Admission neurological examination revealed an awake woman complaining of severe headache and back pain. There was moderate nuchal rigidity. Mental status and cranial nerve testing showed no abnormalities. Motor examination was notable for increased tone in both legs with hyperactive deep tendon reflexes bilaterally. The plantar response was extensor on the left. There was moderate weakness in the left leg. Sensory examination revealed diminished proprioception and vibratory sense in the left leg. There was impairment of pain and temperature sense in the right leg extending to the level of the umbilicus on the right side.

A lumbar puncture showed bloody cerebrospinal fluid confirming the clinical suspicion of subarachnoid hemorrhage. Cerebral angiography was performed which was normal. Myelography revealed widening of the T9-T12 segments of the spinal cord as well as multiple tortuous filling defects on the dorsal surface of the spinal cord which were consistent with abnormally large blood vessels. Selective spinal angiography showed a spinal cord arteriovenous malformation supplied by T9-T11 radicular arteries on the left side. There were both intra- and extramedullary components of the malformation. A large venous aneurysm was also seen.

NEUROANATOMICAL CLUE: Clinical localization of lesions involving the spinal cord depend on a detailed understanding of three longitudinally coursing spinal tracts. These include the <u>uncrossed</u> lateral corticospinal tracts and posterior columns and the <u>crossed</u> spinothalamic tracts.

Spinal Angiogram:

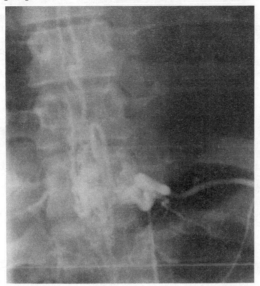

Figure 8.1

QUESTIONS:

1. Based on the neurological examination give the appropriate level and location of the lesion within the spinal cord.

2. Why was cerebral angiography performed in this patient?

3. What diagnostic studies are the most useful in establishing the diagnosis of spinal cord arteriovenous malformation (AVM)?

4. List the three basic types of spinal AVMs. Include the age and sex distribution as well as the clinical features of each type of AVM.

5. What are the therapeutic modalities currently available for the treatment of these lesion?

ANSWERS:

1. This patient demonstrates a <u>Brown-Séquard syndrome</u> involving the left side of the spinal cord. There is ipsilateral posterior column dysfunction manifested by diminished proprioception and vibratory sense in the left leg. The left corticospinal tract is also affected, producing increased tone, a pathological plantar response, and weakness of the left leg. Spasticity in the right leg suggests dysfunction of the right corticospinal tract. The corticospinal tracts are particularly sensitive to compression and thus may be affected bilaterally even when lesions are located on one side of the spinal cord. The <u>crossed</u> nature of the spinothalamic tracts is responsible for the decreased temperature and pain perception on the right side.

   Localization of the level of thoracic spinal cord pathology can most accurately be estimated by defining the level of pain and temperature loss. Because the fibers conveying these sensory modalities for each dermatome cross obliquely in a cephalad direction to the contralateral spinothalamic tract, there will be sparing of one or two dermatomal segments. Thus, although the loss of pain and temperature sense was localized to the T10 dermatome the actual level of the spinal AVM was the T8-T9 cord segment.

2. In the absence of trauma, <u>the most common cause of subarachnoid hemorrhage in the adult population is rupture of a cerebral aneurysm</u>. Cerebral angiography is the procedure of choice in identifying aneurysms. In this patient, the presence of findings localized to the thoracic level of the spinal cord indicate the possibility of a thoracic lesion but cerebral angiography is necessary to exclude an aneurysm, which is a far more common cause of subarachnoid hemorrhage.

3. Myelography, utilizing a water-soluble contrast agent, is currently the most useful screening test in identifying the presence of spinal AVMs. It will identify the lesion in about 90% of patients with spinal AVMs. The typical appearance on myelography is single or multiple serpiginous filling defects located on the surface of the spinal cord. These defects represent enlarged feeding arteries or draining veins. Recent experience with magnetic resonance imaging (MRI) of spinal AVMs suggests that MRI may ultimately replace myelography as a screening procedure. Selective spinal angiography is required in every patient suspected of harboring a spinal AVM. Individual catheterization of all radicular arteries allows the precise identification of all arterial feeders to the malformation. This information is vital in planning any surgical or embolic therapy.

4. Spinal cord AVMs are relatively rare lesions. Spinal tumors are about 20 times more common. Despite their rarity, there are an unusually large number of eponyms ascribed to these lesions. The most common type of spinal AVM is the long dorsal AVM which is also called Type I or angioma racemosum venosum. Recent evidence suggests that this type of AVM, which accounts for 60 to 80% of all spinal AVMs, may represent an acquired fistulous communication between a dural branch of a radicular artery and a dural vein. This transdural fistula is usually located in the dural root sleeve near the dorsal root ganglion. Because there are no valves at this level of the spinal venous system, arterial blood at an increased pressure travels retrogradely from the dura into the posterior spinal veins located on the dorsal surface of the spinal cord. The resulting venous hypertension produces spinal cord ischemia because of a decrease in spinal cord perfusion pressure. This type of malformation is much more common in men and usually produces symptoms after the age of 40 years. The majority are located in the lower thoracic region. The typical clinical syndrome is generally a gradually progressive myelopathy which may be present for several years before diagnosis.

Step-like exacerbation of symptoms, suggesting
acute venous thrombosis, may also occur.
Subarachnoid hemorrhage is distinctly unusual with
these lesions.

The second type of spinal AVM are true AVMs
which are congenital lesions resulting from
abnormal development of the spinal vascular system.
They are structurally similar to the AVMs found
intracranially. These AVMs occur about equally in
men and women and usually produce symptoms in the
second and third decades of life. They are more
common in the cervical region and in the area of
the conus medullaris. The onset of symptoms is
usually acute resulting from an intramedullary or
subarachnoid hemorrhage. Venous thrombosis may also
be responsible for an acute presentation. A more
slowly progressive myelopathy, produced by a
vascular steal phenomena, may also occur.
Angiographically, these AVMs demonstrate high flow
through an arteriovenous shunt. The arterial feeder
may be single but, more commonly, there are
multiple feeding vessels. Venous aneurysms are
present in about 30% of cases. These AVMs may be
entirely intramedullary, both intra- and
extramedullary, or entirely extramedullary. The
majority have at least some intramedullary
component. Subcategories of this type of AVM
include the GLOMUS and JUVENILE malformations.

The third type of spinal AVM consists of a
single fistulous communication between the anterior
spinal artery and vein. This type of AVM is quite
rare and may produce symptoms from hemorrhage or
vascular steal.

5.   The goal of treatment is complete obliteration of
the abnormal shunt because the natural history of
untreated spinal AVMs is generally neurological
devastation either from a progressive myelopathy or
repeated hemorrhage. In most cases obliteration of
the shunt can be achieved surgically. For Type I
AVMs simple ligation of the draining vein or
excision of the dural fistula is the most effective
treatment. Type II and Type III AVMs can usually
also be effectively treated by excision of the

arteriovenous shunt. If, however, the AVM extends
over multiple cord segments, involves the entire
tranverse diameter of the spinal cord, or has
extensive venous drainage, surgical excision may
not be possible. In these cases, transvascular
embolization, using either silastic pellets or
calibrated polyvinyl alcohol particles, may be more
appropriate. The risk of embolization is
inadvertent occlusion of normal arteries to the
spinal cord from stray emboli. This is
particularly true when the AVM is supplied by
branches from the anterior spinal artery. Recent
advances in catheter technology, including the
ability to selectively pass tiny cathoters for
long distances within the anterior spinal artery,
are allowing more aggressive interventional
radiological approaches to these lesions.

PEARLS:

1. Up to 20% of true spinal AVMs will be associated
    with cutaneous vascular anomalies which usually
    correspond to the same metameric distribution as
    the spinal AVM. These cutaneous lesions are
    generally in the form of discrete vascular nevi,
    but extensive nevi associated with enlargement of
    an entire limb (Klippel-Trenaunay-Weber syndrome)
    may also occur.

2. A detailed understanding of the vascular supply to
    the spinal cord is essential before attempting any
    type of therapeutic intervention. The vascular
    supply to the spinal cord has already been outlined
    in the section on spinal cord tumors.

    In general, the penetrating arteries of the
    spinal cord are functionally end-arteries and
    occlusion of these vessels will usually produce
    neurological deficits. The effect of occlusion of
    the larger radicular arteries is variable and
    depends on the extent of collateral circulation.
    Although major radicular arteries, including the
    artery of Adamkiewicz, may occasionally be
    sacrificed without producing neurological deficits,
    occlusion of these vessels should be avoided. This
    is particularly true in the midthoracic region
    where collateral circulation is precarious.

PITFALLS:

1. Early diagnosis of patients with spinal AVMs is essential. Patients treated early in the course of their disease, when they are neurologically normal or have only minor neurological deficits, have the best outcomes. Conversely, the patients who have significant neurological deficits, particularly if their deficits have been progressive over a long period, usually recover very little function after obliteration of the AVM.

2. Partial obliteration of the AVM either from ligation of feeding vessels or embolization is inadequate. Although patients may improve following partial treatment, they remain at risk for future neurological devastation from an incompletely treated AVM.

REFERENCES

1. Aminoff MJ, Barnard RO, Logue V: The pathophysiology of spinal vascular malformations. J Neurol Sci 23:255-263, 1974.

2. Dichiro G, Werner L: Angiography of the spinal cord. A review of contemporary techniques and applications. J Neurosurg 39:1-29, 1973.

3. Kendall BE, Logue V: Spinal epidural angiomatous malformations draining into intrathecal veins. Neuroradiology 13:181-189, 1977.

4. Logue V: Angiomas of the spinal cord: review of the pathogenesis, clinical features and results of surgery. J Neurol Neurosurg Psychiatry 42:1-11, 1979.

5. Malis LI: Arteriovenous malformations of the spinal cord. In Youmans JR, ed. Neurological surgery, Philadelphia, Saunders, 1982, pp 1850-1874.

6. Oldfield EM, Dichiro G, Quindlen EA, et al: Successful treatment of a group of spinal cord arteriovenous malformations by interruption of dural fistula. J Neurosurg 59:1019-1030, 1983.

AMENORRHEA, GALACTORRHEA, AND VISUAL DISTURBANCE

CASE 9: This 22-year-old woman had normal menstrual periods for 5 years following menarche at age 13. Shortly after her 18th birthday, however, her menstrual periods became irregular and were associated with headaches. Subsequently, she ceased having periods altogether and developed mild galactorrhea. She denied changes in her libido or hirsutism. Her headaches, centered behind both eyes, also increased in frequency and severity. She also noted bumping into things while walking and difficulty seeing cars to both the left and right while driving.

Her general examination was significant only for mild obesity and glacatorrhea. There was no hirsutism or skin changes. Pelvic examination was normal. Neurologically her visual acuity was 20/40 in the right eye and 20/60 in the left eye. She demonstrated a bitemporal hemianopsia to confrontational testing. Fundi were normal. The remainder of her neurological examination was unremarkable. A prolactin level measured 600 ng/ml.

Neuroanatomical Clue:

The relationship of the optic chiasm to the pituitary gland results in the characteristic bitemporal field loss associated with pituitary lesions.

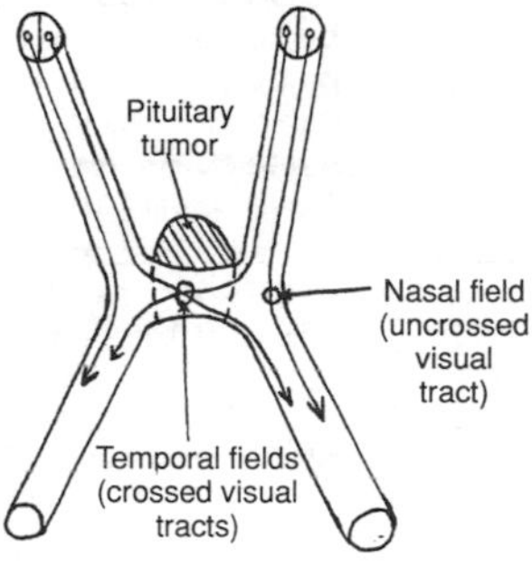

Figure 9.1

QUESTIONS:

1. Describe the major categories of pituitary adenomas and their associated clinical syndromes.

2. What radiologic tests are especially useful in the diagnosis of pituitary adenomas?

3. What laboratory test are most helpful in evaluation of secretory adenomas?

4. How are pituitary adenomas treated?

ANSWERS:

1. Pituitary adenomas may be classified by size. Those tumors <u>less than 1 cm in diameter are considered microadenomas</u>; larger tumors are macroadenomas.

    In the past, pituitary adenomas were further classified by simple staining techniques as <u>chromophobic, basophilic, or acidophilic</u>. Although acromegaly was commonly associated with acidophilic tumors and Cushing's disease with basophilic ones, precise functional classification was possible only with the development of more sophisticated immunocytochemical and ultrastructural techniques.

    Currently pituitary adenomas may be divided into 2 broad categories: <u>nonfunctional and hypersecretory</u>. The latter category may be further subdivided into 7 types. Prolactin secreting tumors are most common and account for 30-70% of pituitary adenomas in men and women. In women they classically present with amenorrhea-galactorrhea syndrome as in this case. Primary amenorrhea is less common than cessation of menstruation following normal menarche. Men more commonly present with headache, visual changes, and impotence. Galactorrhea in men is unusual.

    <u>Somatotrophic adenomas</u> result in 2 clinical syndromes, depending on the age of occurrence. <u>Gigantism</u> occurs when this tumor arises in young patients prior to closure of the epiphyseal plates of the long bones. Pituitary gigantism is rare. Older patients develop characteristic <u>acromegalic features </u>including coarse facial features with prognathism and macroglossia and enlargement of the hands and feet. These result from bony overgrowth and thickening of the soft tissue and skin. The altered physical appearance is frequently accompanied by headache (50-75% of patients), arthralgias, and lethargy. Cardiac disease and abnormal carbohydrate metabolism also occur. Because of their insidious changes, diagnosis of growth hormone secreting tumors is often delayed. Overall growth hormone adenomas comprise about 15-25% of pituitary adenomas.

Cushing's disease results from ACTH-secreting adenomas and represent about 5% of pituitary adenomas. The well-known clinical features of this syndrome, mostly due to excess secretion of glucocorticoids, include truncal obesity, moon facies, striae, hirsutism, easy bruising from skin and capillary fragility, poor wound healing, glucose intolerance, hypertension, and osteoporosis. Oligomenorrhea, amenorrhea, or impotence is present in 70-80% of patients. A proximal myopathy is also common.

Thyroid-stimulating hormone-secreting adenomas, which present with clinical features of hyperthyroidism, and gonadotropic adenomas are rare. Stem cell adenomas and mixed secreting adenomas account for less than 5% of pituitary adenomas.

Finally, 20-25% of pituitary adenomas are endocrinologically nonfunctional. These null cell adenomas may be further classified as oncocytic or nononcocytic. Because these tumors do not secrete hormones, they frequently are not detected until large in size, often extending beyond the sella, with symptoms referable to the mass itself. A recent review of these tumors revealed 72 of 100 patients presented with visual loss, 61 had symptoms of hypopituitarism, and 36 had headache.

2. Plain skull x-rays are still useful in the evaluation of pituitary adenomas. Abnormalities that should be looked for include enlargement of the sella, thinning of the dorsum sella, erosion of the floor or loss of the lamina dura forming the floor, elevation or erosion of the anterior clinoid processes, or a true double floor.

Computed tomography (CT) scanning has greatly enhanced diagnostic capabilities. Pre- and postcontrast series should be obtained including axial and coronal views of the sella. Microadenomas of only 3-4 mm in diameter may now be seen as hypodense lesions within the pituitary gland. Increased height of the gland, exceeding

9 mm, may also indicate the presence of tumor.   In larger lesions erosion of the sella may also be seen.   The intra- and suprasellar extent of macroadenomas can be accurately defined as can the relationship of the tumor to the pituitary stalk and optic chiasm.   Magnetic resonance imaging is also useful in this regard and offers the advantage of exceptional sagittal views of this region. Adenomas are usually of low signal intensity on T-1 weighted images and high intensity on T-2.

3.   The most important laboratory test in evaluation of a suspected prolactin secreting adenoma is the basal serum prolactin level, which ranges from 5-20 ng/ml in normal individuals.   A prolactin level of 50 ng/ml is associated with the presence of a prolactinoma in approximately 25% of patients. When this level rises to 100 ng/ml, a prolactinoma can be found in nearly 50% of patients and a level of 200-300 ng/ml virtually assures the presence of such a tumor (100%).   Mild elevations in prolactin (< 200 ng/ml) may also result from lesions that compromise the pituitary stalk, subsequently diminishing the normal dopamine inhibition of prolactin secretion.

Growth hormone is normally present in the serum at levels of 2-5 ng/ml.   Elevations greater than 10 ng/ml are usually indicative of somatotropic adenomas.

In Cushing's disease the plasma cortisol level is generally elevated although wide variability limits the usefulness of isolated plasma values. The loss of normal diurnal variation in plasma cortisol levels is more helpful in diagnosis as is quantitation of 24 hour urine free cortisol and 17-OH corticosteroids.   Direct measurement of plasma ACTH is generally not helpful.   Most critically, in Cushing's disease cortisol levels are not suppressed by low dose dexamethasone [0.5 mg 4 times daily (qid) for 2 days] but are suppressed by high dose dexamethasone (2 mg qid for 2 days, 4 times daily) to less than 50% of baseline values.   Non-suppression with high dose dexamethasone, elevated cortisol, and abnormally low

ACTH levels in the blood areindicative of an
adrenal tumor or hyperplasia rather than an ACTH
secreting pituitary adenoma.

Finally, in large adenomas compression of the
gland may lead to multiple endocrinopathies.
Baseline thyroid function tests, follicle-
stimulating hormone, luteinizing hormone, cortisol,
and prolactin levels should be obtained.

4. Nonfunctional pituitary adenomas, as noted above,
    generally present as large masses. The surgical
    indications are relatively straightforward and
    include progressive visual loss whether acuity or
    fields, dysfunction of cranial nerves III, IV, or
    VI, increased intracranial pressure from local mass
    effect, cerebrospinal fluid (CSF) obstruction and
    hydrocephalus, pituitary apoplexy, and CSF leak.
    Medical therapy has not proved beneficial.
    Radiation therapy is offered to patients when tumor
    resection is not complete.

    In functioning adenomas, surgery remains the
    treatment of choice for patients with Cushing's
    disease, acromegaly, or Nelson's syndrome. The
    decision is more complex regarding prolactinomas.
    Bromocriptine has been demonstrated to normalize
    serum prolactin levels in patients with both micro
    and macroadenomas. Furthermore, actual shrinkage
    of tumor size has been documented even in large
    tumors. Therefore, many physicians consider
    bromocriptine the initial treatment of choice in
    prolactin secreting tumors, especially in view of
    its very limited adverse effects. Selective
    transphenoidal adenectomy has been shown to have a
    lower recurrence rate in microdenomas, however, and
    may still be recommended as a first line therapy,
    especially in women of childbearing years. Some
    patients simply do not tolerate bromocriptine, even
    in low doses and surgery is then an excellent
    alternative. Patients who desire pregnancy are
    often treated surgically but some cases have been
    managed medically as well, with very close followup
    throughout the pregnancy. In these instances, the
    choice of surgical or medical management must be

carefully individualized for each patient. In prolactinomas that demonstrate progressive growth despite an adequate trial of medical therapy or in the presence of progressive visual loss, apoplexy, oculomotor dysfunction, hydrocephalus or elevated intracranial pressure, surgery is clearly indicated.

Microadenomas are approached via the transphenoidal route as repopularized by Hardy. Even most macroadenomas may be approached transphenoidally as much of the tumor will drop into the sella as the operation proceeds. Significant extension anteriorly beneath the frontal lobes or laterally into the middle fossa may necessitate transcranial operation. This operation, however, has higher morbidity and mortality than the transphenoidal route, including a significant risk of making vision worse.

Supervoltage radiation therapy has been shown to improve recurrence free rates. Indications include significant residual tumor on CT after surgery, surgical failures (recurrence of tumor or hypersecretory state), and large tumors that cannot be safely and totally resected.

PEARLS:

1.   Pituitary adenomas are exceptionally common and have been reported in 20-23% of all pituitary glands in large autopsy series. In clinical series approximately 35% of adenomas are invasive (but not malignant).

2.   Pituitary apoplexy is used in several ways by different authors but Cushing originally used this term to describe hemorrhage into an adenoma. Infarction with swelling can produce a similar clinical picture which consists of headache, sudden deterioration of vision and/or oculomotor palsies, and acute hypopituitarism.

PITFALLS:

1. Carotid artery aneurysms may present as intrasellar
    masses and have been mistaken for pituitary
    adenomas. Transphenoidal operation with aneurysmal
    rupture and death have occurred. Arteriography is
    usually diagnostic.

2. Although adenomas are the most common lesions in
    the sellar and suprasellar area, many others can
    occur there, mimicking an adenoma, and should be
    considered. These include craniopharyngioma;
    arachnoid, epidermoid and Rathke's cleft cysts,
    hamartomas; dermoids and epidermoids, gliomas,
    meningiomas, and metastatic tumors.

REFERENCES

1. Black PM, Zervas NT, Ridgeway EC, Martin JB:
   Secretory tumors of the pituitary gland. New York,
   Raven Press, 1984.

2. Ebersold MJ, Quast LM, Laws ER, Scheithauer B,
   Randall RV: Long term results in transphenoidal
   removal of nonfunctioning pituitary adenomas. J
   Neurosurg 64:13-719, 1986.

3. Post KD, Biller BJ, Adelman LS, Molitch ME, Wolpert
   SM, Reichlin S: Selective transphenoidal
   adenomectomy in women with galactorrhea-
   amenorrhea. JAMA 242:158-162, 1979.

4. Post KD, Jackson IM, Reinchlin S eds: The
   pituitary adenoma. New York, Plenum, 1980.

5. Post KD, Muraszko K: Management of pituitary tumors.
   Neurologic Clinics 4:801-831, 1987.

6. Scheithauer BW, Kovacs KT, Laws ER, Randall RV:
   Pathology of invasive pituitary tumors with special
   reference to functional classification. J Neurosurg
   65:733-744, 1986.

7. Wilson CB, Dempsey LC: Transphenoidal microsurgical
   removal of 250 pituitary adenomas. J Neurosurg 48:
   13-22, 1978.

BLUNT HEAD TRAUMA WITH BRIEF LOSS OF CONSCIOUSNESS FOLLOWED BY TRANSIENT TETRAPLEGIA

CASE 10:   A 19-year-old woman sustained blunt head trauma by striking her head on the bottom of a pool in a diving accident. Witnesses reported a brief period of unconsciousness during which time she was brought out of the pool by alert lifeguards. Upon regaining consciousness the patient complained of total paralysis of her arms and legs and numbness of her entire body below the neck. On transfer to the hospital she noted some movement in her arms. Cognitive function was intact and there were no cranial nerve abnormalities. Motor examination was notable for complete paralysis of the biceps, brachioradialis, supinator, and pronator muscles bilaterally. There was mild weakness of both triceps muscles.

A lateral cervical spine x-ray revealed a burst fracture of the C5 vertebra. There was loss of height of the body of the vertebra and posterior displacement of a bony fragment into the spinal canal. There was a widened distance between the spinous processes of C5 and C6.

Initial treatment consisted of external immobilization of the cervical spine with a halo ring and 15 pounds of cervical traction. Over the next 48 hours the patient had almost complete return of neurological function in her arms. On hospital day 4 she underwent internal stabilization through an anterior cervical approach with resection of the C5 vertebral body and an interbody fusion with an iliac bone graft. She made a complete recovery.

CLUE:

A cervical spine injury should be suspected in any patient who has sustained significant head injury. In this patient the appearance of transient tetraplegia without respiratory compromise suggested that the level of the injury was below the C4 spinal segment. The persistence of the C6 and C7 radicular dysfunction further pointed to a fracture of the lower cervical spine.

QUESTIONS:

1. Describe the radiographic features and mechanism of injury of a cervical spine burst fracture.

2. What was the rationale for the application of cervical traction in this patient?

3. Discuss the initial management of a patient with a cervical spine fracture.

4. What are the indications for emergency operative treatment of cervical spine fractures?

ANSWERS:

1. A burst, or compression, fracture describes a
    comminuted fracture of a vertebral body. The
    radiographic features of a burst fracture vary
    according to the severity of the injury. The least
    severe form will appear simply as a loss of height
    of the fractured vertebral body on lateral
    radiograph. This form of a compression fracture is
    considered stable and may be managed conservatively
    with a hard collar. A more severe injury will
    actually shatter the vertebral body and may produce
    spinal cord injury from posterior displacement of
    bony fragments into the spinal canal. Frequently,
    there will be associated injuries to the posterior
    elements such as a fracture of the neural arch or
    disruption of the interspinous ligaments. When
    there are associated injuries to the posterior
    elements then the burst fracture should be
    considered an unstable injury and external skeletal
    immobilization with a halo ring or tongs should be
    applied. The increased distance between the C5 and
    C6 spinous processes in this patient was consistent
    with a tear of the interspinous ligament at this
    level and, thus, her fracture was considered
    unstable.

    The mechanism of injury producing this type of
    fracture is either an axial loading force applied
    to the vertex of the head or a forced flexion
    injury.

2. There are several indications for the application
    of cervical traction in the initial management of
    cervical spine injuries. These include:
    1) immobilization of the cervical spine in patients
    with unstable fractures 2) reduction of
    dislocations or subluxations 3) distraction of the
    intervertebral foramina in patients with radicular
    compression and 4) alleviation of pain produced by
    associated soft tissue injury.

    In this patient the unstable nature of her
    fracture as well as the clinical evidence of nerve
    root compression were the indications for the
    application of cervical traction.

3. The primary goal of the initial emergency management of patients with cervical spine fractures and dislocations is to <u>prevent secondary injury</u> to either the spinal cord or nerve roots. This is important even in patients who have suffered immediate functional spinal cord transection at the level of the fracture. Preservation of even a single cord segment above the level of injury can make a vast difference in the long-term rehabilitation of a patient with permanent spinal cord injury.

   Immobilization of the neck during the initial resuscitation or medical evaluation of the trauma patient is crucial. This is frequently overlooked in the acutely ill patient with multiple injuries and unstable vital signs. Emergency medical technicians are trained to immobilize the neck of patients sustaining significant trauma. A sandbag or a hard cervical collar is the usual type of immobilization applied at the scene of the injury. Whatever the form of immobilization employed it should be kept in place until the cervical spine can be evaluated by a lateral radiograph. Once a cervical spine fracture has been identified the stability of the fracture must be assessed. Any patient with a cervical spine fracture which is considered unstable should immediately be placed in external skeletal fixation and traction with either a halo ring or tongs. The amount of traction suspended from the fixation device varies but, as a general rule, the initial amount of traction should be calculated at 3-5 pounds per cervical vertebrae. Thus, 15-25 pounds of cervical traction should initially be applied for an unstable C5 fracture. If repeat x-ray shows incomplete reduction of a displaced fracture or subluxation then additional weight should be added in slow increments until the fracture-dislocation is reduced. In the majority of cervical spine fractures and dislocations the cervical spine can be effectively immobilized and reduced with external skeletal fixation and traction.

4.   There are 2 clear indications for emergency surgical management of cervical spine fractures and dislocations. These indications are: <u>1) a progressive neurological deficit and 2) the presence of an incomplete spinal cord injury</u>. In both instances surgery should only be performed if there is evidence of extrinsic compression of the spinal cord obtained at myelography. Emergency surgical intervention for stabilization or reduction is seldom necessary because this can generally be achieved with skeletal traction.

Although there are reports of significant neurological recovery in patients with complete loss of neurological function below the level of injury who are decompressed surgically within 24 hours of their injury, it is generally not believed that emergent surgical intervention is always necessary in patients who exhibit immediate and complete loss of neurological function below the level of their fracture at the time of injury.

PEARLS:

1.   Injuries to the cervical spine are traditionally divided into upper and lower cervical spine fractures and dislocations. Injuries to the upper spine include fractures and dislocations involving the base of the occiput through C2. Injuries at this level occur infrequently in the adult, representing less than 25% of fractures and dislocations of the cervical spine. In the pediatric population, however, the majority of cervical spine injuries involve the upper level.

Injuries to the lower cervical spine include fractures and dislocations involving the C3 through C7 vertebrae.   <u>The C5 vertebra is the most commonly fractured vertebra</u>. Injuries to the lower cervical spine are more likely to be associated with a spinal cord injury probably because the ratio of the cross-sectional areas of the spinal canal to the spinal cord is less in the lower cervical spine than in the upper cervical spine.

2. <u>An important clue to the presence and severity of a</u>
    <u>cervical spine injury is widening of the</u>
    <u>prevertebral soft tissue space</u>. Significant injury
    and instability may exist in the absence of any
    obvious bony abnormality on plain films. In these
    cases, the only evidence of injury may be a widened
    retropharyngeal or retrotracheal space.

    The retropharyngeal space extends from the
    posterior margin of the pharyngeal air shadow to
    the anteroinferior aspect of the axis. A
    measurement greater than 7 mm is abnormal. The
    retrotracheal space is defined as the soft tissue
    space between the posterior limit of the tracheal
    air shadow to the anteroinferior aspect of the C6
    vertebral body. Although this space varies
    considerably with age and respiration measurements
    greater than 14 mm in children and 22 mm in the
    adult are considered abnormal, a significant
    cervical spine injury should be suspected.

PITFALLS:

1. <u>It is important to visualize all cervical vertebrae</u>
    <u>on the lateral radiograph</u> in patients sustaining
    significant trauma. Frequently, the initial x-ray
    will not adequately visualize C7 because of the
    overlying shoulders. Irreversible spinal cord
    damage has secondarily resulted from neck
    manipulation in patients with unstable C7 fractures
    or dislocations in which C7 was not visualized on
    the initial cervical spine film.

2. Excessive neck manipulation has also resulted in
    permanent spinal cord injury during the initial
    resuscitation of a trauma patient. Although
    maintenance of an airway is vital, <u>excessive</u>
    <u>extension of the neck for intubation before a</u>
    <u>cervical fracture is ruled out must be avoided</u>. If
    an artificial airway is required before a cervical
    spine film can be obtained then either an emergency
    cricothyroidotomy or nasal intubation should be
    performed.

REFERENCES

1. Apuzzo MLJ, Heiden JS, Weiss MH, et al: Acute fractures of the odontoid process. J Neurosurg 48:85-91, 1978.

2. Bohlman HH: Acute fractures and dislocations of the cervical spine: An analysis of 300 hospitalized patients and review of the literature. J Bone Joint Surg 61A:1119-1142, 1979.

3. Holdworth FW: Fractures, dislocations, and fracture-dislocations of the spine. J Bone Joint Surg 52A:1534-1551, 1970.

4. Whitley JF, Forsyth HF: Classification of cervical spine injuries. Am J Roentgenol 83:633-644, 1960.

VISUAL LOSS AND THIRD NERVE PALSY

CASE 11: A previously healthy 47-year-old woman was evaluated for poor vision in her right eye that was first noticed when she closed her left eye and discovered she could not see from her right eye. Fundospopic examination revealed right optic nerve pallor and visual fields demonstrated a central scotoma (blindspot) in this eye with a small junctional scotoma in the upper outer quadrant in her left eye. A third nerve palsy of her right eye was also detected and the rest of the examination was within normal limits. A computed tomography (CT) scan was performed and revealed a large contrast enhancing mass in the region of the right cavernous sinus. This was followed by an anqiogram which was diagnostic.

Neuroanatomic Clue:

Angiogram

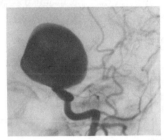

Figure 11.1

QUESTIONS:

1. Given the visual field findings, which portion of the visual system is affected by this lesion: orbital optic nerve, intracranial optic nerve, optic chiasm, or optic tract? What is the anatomical basis of these defects?

2. What is the diagnosis and definition of this lesion?

3. What other lesions can produce similar physical findings?

4. What is the natural history of this lesion and what other locations in the central nervous system (CNS) does this lesion occur?

5. What treatments can be offered to this patient?

ANSWERS:

1. <u>Intracranial optic nerve</u> - This lesion demonstrates
    the effects of chronic compression of the
    intracranial optic nerve. The most sensitive
    portion of the optic nerve to extrinsic compression
    is the <u>papillomacular bundle conveying retinal</u>
    <u>nerve fibers of the central visual field</u>. This
    compression has resulted in a central scotoma in
    the affected eye and the chronic nature of this
    compression is reflected by the optic atrophy seen
    on fundoscopic examination of the retina. Although
    noncompressive causes of optic atrophy and central
    scotoma are possible, the additional findings of a
    IIIrd nerve palsy and a <u>contralateral junction</u>
    <u>scotoma</u> point to an extrinsic compressive etiology.
    The visual defect in the opposite eye results from
    the descussating fibers of the nasal portion of the
    left retina which loop forward into the right optic
    nerve before joining the right temporal retinal
    fibers to form the right optic tract. As the
    fibers in the nasal portion of the left retina
    subserve vision in the temporal field of the left
    eye, compression of the right intracranial portion
    of the optic nerve can produce a temporal visual
    deficit in the opposite eye thus confirming the
    diagnosis of intracranial optic nerve compression.
    In all cases of visual loss in one eye it is
    essential to check for a junctional scotoma in the
    opposite eye and the function of the cranial nerves
    which are in anatomical juxtaposition to the
    intracranial visual system in the region of the
    cavernous sinus (III, IV, V, VI). The combination
    of the above symptoms should always indicate the
    need for a CT scan in such a patient.

2. The angiogram reveals the presence of a large
    <u>aneurysm of the proximal internal carotid artery</u>
    near the origin of the ophthalmic artery. Because
    this aneurysm is greater than 2.5 cm in diameter,
    it is classified as a giant aneurysm. Anatomically
    it is important to remember that the first major
    intracranial branch of the carotid artery as it
    leaves the cavernous sinus and enters the

subarachnoid space of the brain is the <u>ophthalmic artery</u>. The following branches are the posterior communicating artery and the anterior choroidal artery after which the carotid artery bifurcates into the anterior and middle cerebral arteries.

3. Lesions resulting in the compression of the intracranial optic nerve or chiasm and the cranial nerves in the region of the cavernous sinus include meningiomas, aneurysms, metastatic lesions, inflammatory conditions of the superior orbital fissure, pituitary tumors, craniopharyngiomas, chordomas, or thrombosis of the cavernous sinus.

4. <u>Approximately 5% of all intracranial aneurysms are giant in size</u>. Although these aneurysms may occur in any location within the brain, they are most frequently found in the following locations; internal carotid artery (cavernous and ophthalmic portions); middle cerebral artery (bifurcation most commonly); vertobasilar system (top of basilar): anterior cerebral artery (communicating portion). These aneurysms present in all age groups but are most frequently symptomatic between the ages of 30 and 60 years and affect women 2 times as commonly as men. The natural history of giant aneurysms is not completely known. Approximately 30% of patients harboring such an aneurysm will present with a subarachnoid hemorrhage that is identical in symptomatology to bleeds from smaller aneurysms. Because of the large size of these aneurysms and their tendency to increase in size or partially thrombose with time, the remaining symptomatic patients will present with physical signs referable to the location in the brain of the aneurysm. Because of the great frequency of these aneurysms in the anterior portion of the circulation of the brain, 80% of patients will have signs of optic, oculomotor, or abducens nerve compression. It is now believed that giant aneurysms bleed as frequently as smaller aneurysms, probably at the rate of 3% per year. The prognosis is grave with <u>80% of symptomatic patients dead or severely disabled at 5 years</u> from the time of their diagnosis. The diagnosis is usually confirmed by CT and angiography which reveal the presence of a

large homogeneously enhancing intracranial mass in communication with the vascular system. Frequently the CT scan shows a larger lesion than the angiogram as over one-third of these aneurysms are partially thrombosed and therefore incompletely fill during angiography.

5.   Treatment of giant aneurysms is both complex and hazardous. The approach to these lesions is generally defined by their location, size, and particular cerebrovascular anatomy. The preferred treatment when the aneurysm is projecting into the subarachnoid space or brain is direct clipping of the aneurysm neck and preservation of the parent artery when possible. When clipping cannot be achieved, alternatives include the following:

   a)   proximal artery ligation, usually of the common or internal carotid artery;

   b)   entrapment of the aneurysm with occlusion of the proximal artery (usually internal or common carotid) and occlusion of the intracranial vessel immediately distal to the aneurysm. This technique frequently requires a bypass operation to provide blood supply to the vessels distal to the aneurysm such as a superficial temporal artery to middle cerebral artery bypass.

   c)   intravascular procedures such as balloon embolization or wire thrombosis.

PEARLS:

1. Approximately 20% of giant aneurysms will show curvilinear calcium deposits in the aneurysm wall or clot on plain skull films.

2. Giant aneurysms occur with a proportionally increased frequency in children compared with adults.

3. Partial thrombosis of a giant aneurysm does not protect against future subarachnoid hemorrhage from the aneurysm.

4. Six percent of giant aneurysms are greater than 3 cm in diameter.

5. Fifty percent of vertebral-basilar aneurysms present with subarachnoid hemorrhage.

6. Giant aneurysms may be larger than angiography indicates as the aneurysm may be filled with clotted blood. CT scan or magnetic resonance imaging (MRI) will reveal the true dimensions of the aneurysm as the thrombosed portion is readily visualized.

PITFALLS:

1. Giant aneurysms may mimic the CT appearance of tumors, abscesses, or intracerebral hemorrhages by producing a "ring sign" or appearance on the contrast study.

2. Thrombosis of a giant aneurysm may be associated with significant edema and mass effect on the brain causing an abrupt clinical deterioration without the presence of a subarachnoid hemorrhage.

3. Because of their size and proximity to cerebrospinal fluid (CSF) outflow pathways (particularly in the posterior fossa), giant aneurysms can present with an obstructive hydrocephalus.

4. Large subfrontal extensions of anterior circulation giant aneurysms can cause an organic mental syndrome by frontal lobe compression.

5. Emboli from partially thrombosed giant aneurysms can occur and may mimic the symptoms of a stroke or transient ischemic attack (TIA).

REFERENCES

1. Drake CG: Giant Intracranial aneurysms: experience with surgical treatment in 174 patients. Clin Neurosurg 26:12-95, 1979.

2. Pia HW, Ziersa J: Giant cerebral aneurysms. Neurosurgery Rev 5:117-148, 1982.

3. Morley TP, Barr HWK: Giant intracranial aneurysms: diagnosis, course, and management. Clin Neurosurg 16:73-94, 1969.

4. Sundt TM Jr.: Surgical technique for giant
   intracranial aneurysm. Neurosurgy Rev 5:161-168,
   1982.

5. Sundt TM, Piepgrass DG: Surgical approach to giant
   intracranial aneurysms: operative experience with 80
   cases. J Neurosurg 51:731-742, 1979.

6. Weir B: Aneurysms affecting the nervous system.
   Baltimore, Williams & Wilkins, 1987, pp 187-208.

HEADACHE, VISUAL OBSCURATIONS, AND PAPILLEDEMA

CASE 12: A 27-year-old woman presented with a 3-month history of headaches. The headaches were described as a sensation of pressure in her forehead. Although they were initially intermittent, they gradually became constant and were worse at night or when bending over. In the 2 weeks prior to admission, she had several episodes of bilateral visual obscurations lasting 10 to 15 seconds, usually precipitated by bending or coughing.

On examamination she was noted to be markedly obese. Fundoscopic examination revealed moderate bilateral papilledema. There was some concentric decrease in her visual fields bilaterally. Visual acuity was 20/50 in the right eye and 20/60 in the left eye. Extraoocular movements were full and there were no motor, sensory, gait, or deep tendon reflex abnormalities.

A computed tomography (CT) scan was obtained which was unremarkable except for a slight decrease in ventricular size. A lumbar puncture revealed an opening pressure of 400 mm H_2O with 2 white blood cell count (WBC) (lymphocytes) and normal protein and glucose. Formal visual field testing showed enlarged blind spots bilaterally in addition to concentric visual field loss.

QUESTIONS:

1. What is your diagnosis?

2. What conditions may cause this disease?

3. What are the treatment considerations?

4. What is the role of surgery for these patients?

5. What follow-up should be provided for these individuals?

71

ANSWERS:

1. The diagnosis of <u>pseudotumor cerebri or benign intracranial hypertension</u> is made in patients with headaches, papilledema and increased intracranial pressure in the absence of central nervous system (CNS) inflammatory disease, venous occlusion or space occupying masses. The pathophysiology of this condition is not well understood but involves a generalized cerebral edema. Pseudotumor is often associated with obesity, pregnancy or menstrual irregularities. Typically it involves women during adolescence or early adulthood.

2. Many other medical disorders have been associated with pseudotumor although most commonly it is idiopathic. <u>Endocrine disorders</u> such as Addison's disease, Cushing's disease, and hypoparathyroidism have been implicated. <u>Drug associations</u> include exogenous steroids, steroid withdrawal, birth control pills, tetracycline, nitrofurantoin, and sulfamethasoxisole. <u>Impaired cerebral venous</u> drainage as in dural sinus thrombosis may cause elevated intracranial pressure. Other etiologies include excess or deficiency of <u>vitamin A, systemic lupus erythematosus and various hematological disorders</u> such as pernicious anemia, iron deficiency anemia, polycythemia vera, and thrombocytopenia.

3. Medical therapy is directed toward preventing the progression of visual symptoms and controlling headache. <u>Prednisone</u> has been found to be effective in this regard. <u>Diuretics</u> such as furosemide, inhibitors of cerebrospinal fluid (CSF) production such as acetazolamide and hyperosmotic agents such as glycerol have also had some success. Acetazolamide, a carbonic anhydrase inhibitor, may have a direct effect on the decreased production of CSF in addition to its diuretic action, and in high doses may be more effective than steroids or furosemide. Weight loss alone can be successful in controlling symptoms. Most patients respond to serial lumbar punctures where varying amounts of CSF are removed. Lumbar punctures may be repeated

daily at first and then at increasing intervals until symptoms and intracranial pressure are controlled.

4. Surgery is reserved for patients who are refractory to medical therapy or serial lumbar punctures, particularly when they have progressive visual impairment. Shunting procedures, either lumboperitoneal or ventriculoperitoneal, are almost always effective in controlling symptoms and pressure. Ventriculoperitoneal shunts tend to malfunction less often than lumbar shunts, however, because the ventricles are not enlarged and placement of the ventricular tubing can be technically difficult. Other surgical treatments include subtemporal decompression and optic nerve decompression by excision of the optic nerve sheath in the orbit.

5. Most cases of pseudotumor are self-limiting or respond readily to one of the above mentioned therapies. Often, however, the intracranial pressure remains elevated despite adequate control of symptoms. Frequent follow-up visual field testing is crucial to prevent visual loss even when headaches have resolved. The recurrence rate is low although rates of 9 to 43% have been quoted.

PEARLS:

1. Pseudotumor may occasionally occur in children. No frequency differences in gender have been found in this age group. Common etiologies include vitamin A therapy for acne and venous sinus thrombosis due to systemic or ear infection.

2. Remember that pseudotumor is a diagnosis of exclusion. In addition to ruling out venous thrombosis or space occupying masses with appropriate radiological studies, one must rule out the previously mentioned endocrinopathies, drug ingestions, and systemic diseases.

PITFALLS:

1.   Although lumbar punctures are safe in patients with
     pseudotumor, one must be wary of performing them as
     a diagnostic procedure in patients with
     papilledema. Papilledema implies elevated
     intracranial pressure. A CT scan must be obtained
     prior to lumbar puncture to avoid herniation in a
     patient harboring a space occupying mass.

2.   Lumboperitoneal shunts, although highly effective
     in treating pseudotumor, have several drawbacks.
     They are difficult to perform in obese patients and
     often malfunction or cause radiculopathy from
     lumbar nerve root compression. In addition, a
     valve system must be used to avoid hypotension
     headaches.

                        REFERENCES

1. Carglow TJ, Corbett J, Goodwin J, et al:
   Controversies in diagnosis and management of
   pseudotumor cerebre. Arch Neurol 44(2):128-129,
   1987.

2. Donaldson JO: Endocrinology of pseudotumor cerebri.
   Neurol Clin 4(4):919-927, 1986.

3. Fishman RA: The pathophysiology of pseudotumor
   cerebri: an unsolved puzzle. Arch Neurol 41 (3):
   257-258, 1984.

4. Johnston I, Paterson A: Benign intracranial
   hypertention: I. Diagnosis and prognosis. Brain
   97:289-300, 1974.

5. Johnston I, Paterson A, Besser M: The treatment of
   benign intracranial hypertension: A review of 134
   cases. Surg Neurol 16:218-224, 1981.

6. Raichle ME, Grubb RL, Phelps ME, Gado MH, Caronna
   JJ: Cerebral hemodynamics and metabolism in
   pseudotumor cerebri. Ann Neurol 4:104-111, 1978.

7. Weisberg LA: Benign intracranial hypertension.
   Medicine 54:197-207, 1975.

FOCAL SEIZURE IN AN ADULT

<u>CASE 13</u>: A 53-year-old man presented to his doctor complaining of a 15-minute episode of involuntary right-hand movements, speech difficulty, and an intense headache without the loss of consciousness. The patient also noted difficulty concentrating at work, frequent forgetfulness, and increasingly severe morning headaches during the past 4 months. Physical examination revealed mild bilateral papilledema, right hemiparesis involving the face more than the limbs, hyperactive right-sided reflexes, and a right Babinski sign. The rest of the physical and neurological evaluation was within normal limits and the patient had a computed tomography (CT) scan.

Clue:

CT scan

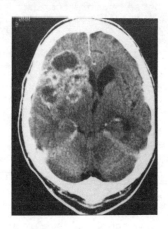

Figure 13.1

QUESTIONS:

1. What is the most likely diagnosis and what would be the differential diagnosis in this case?

2. Is this the typical history for this disease?

3. What is the treatment?

4. What is the prognosis?

ANSWERS:

1. That patient most likely has a primary brain
    tumor known as a <u>grade IV astrocytoma or</u>
    <u>glioblastoma</u>.   The great majority of primary
    supratentorial brain tumors in adults arise from
    glial cell precursors and have been given the name
    of astrocytomas, with pathological gradations of I
    to IV in order of increasing malignancy. The most
    malignant variety astrocytoma grade IV or of
    glioblastoma is unfortunately the most common of
    the group (50%) and has the worst prognosis.
    Although these tumors can arise in any location
    with the central nervous system, they are most
    frequently found in the white matter of the frontal
    or temporal lobes.   They may obtain considerable
    size, undergo rapid growth, and on CT scan show
    evidence of contrast enhancement, edema, and
    displacement of surrounding brain tissue. Although
    the age group, history, examination, and CT scan
    are highly suggestive of the diagnosis of a
    glioblastoma, a biopsy must always be done to
    confirm the grade of the tumor and to exclude other
    pathological conditions which can occasionally
    mimic high grade gliomas.   Such lesions include
    brain <u>abscesses (bacterial, fungal, mycotic),</u>
    <u>metastatic tumors, lymphomas (particularly in</u>
    <u>midline locations), "cryptic" arteriovenous</u>
    <u>malformations (AVMs), sarcomas, and malignant</u>
    <u>meningiomas</u>.   Because the treatment of some of the
    above conditions differs greatly from that of
    glioblastoma, tumor tissue must be obtained prior
    to instituting therapy in these patients.

2. Yes. The characteristic features of the
    glioblastoma in the adult are produced by the
    location of the tumor within the brain, its rapid
    growth potential, and the diffuse effects of
    increased intracranial pressure produced by the
    tumor's mass and edema on the surrounding brain
    tissue.   This leads to a relentless progression of
    the symptoms over a 4- to 6-month period and
    typically results in headaches (particularly in the
    morning), impaired mental functioning, weakness,
    and seizures. Men are affected more commonly than

women, and the frontal and temporal lobes are more frequently involved than the parietal or occipital lobes.

3. Glioblastomas are among the most malignant and refractory tumors to treat in the human body and the therapy of glioblastomas is essentially palliative. Surgery has two objectives: diagnosis and reduction of the mass effect by internal decompression of the tumor. Because of the diffuse and infiltrative nature of this tumor type, total surgical extrapation is rarely possible. The extent of surgical debulking is a function of the clinical status and age of the patient, the size of the lesion, and most importantly the location within the brain. Small polar lesions can be more aggressively treated than large lesions lying within eloquent areas or deep areas of the brain. In some cases, such as the speech area or basal ganglia/thalamus, computer guided stereotaxic biopsy may be preferred to open craniotomy for the diagnosis of these tumors.

Radiation after surgery, usually whole brain with a boost to the tumor bed (4500-6000 rads), has been shown to increase the survival of patients with glioblastoma although the prognosis is still poor. Chemotherapy with nitrosoureas or other multiple agent therapies have not been successful in prolonging survival over 2 years when used in conjunction with aggressive surgery and radiation therapy. Current research suggests that immunological therapy or interstitial irradiation therapy (brachytherapy) with iridium or iodine sources may be beneficial to patients with this refractory and highly aggressive tumor.

4. In patients with glioblastoma, the 1-year survival rate is less than 20% and the 2-year survival rate is less than 10%. Lower grade astrocytomas and oligodendrogliomas have better survival rates particularly if the patient is young and has no other neurological problems save seizures. In certain cases the 10-year survival rate may be over 80% but the majority of patients have a 3- to 5-year life span. The most favorable primary brain

tumor occurs in childhood and is the cystic
cerebellar astrocytoma that is compatible with a
normal life span when complete surgical resection
is accomplished.

PEARLS:

1. Any middle-aged person presenting with their first
   seizure should be presumed to have a brain tumor
   until proven otherwise.

2. Extraneural metastasis from brain tumors is very
   rare but can occur with glioblastoma and usually
   involves the lungs or cervical lymph nodes. Dural
   sinus invasion by the tumor is generally detected in
   these cases.

3. Calcium deposits occur more frequently in
   oligodendrogliomas (60%) and low grade astrocytomas
   (15%) than in glioblastomas (5%). Because of the
   greater prevalence of glioblastomas, however,
   calcium deposits in diagnostic studies of primary
   brain tumors should always include glioblastoma in
   the differential.

4. Seizures occur more frequently in patients with
   oligodendrogliomas and low grade astrocytomas than
   in patients with glioblastomas.

5. Glioblastomas are multifocal in 5 to 10% of cases.

6. The corpus callosum is a frequent site for deep
   glioblastomas and this route allows extensive
   infiltration of both hemispheres. The pathological
   appearance of these particular tumors has led to
   the designation of the term "butterfly glioma" in
   this condition.

7. Patients with neurofibromatosis have a greatly
   increased incidence of primary brain tumors,
   especially gliomas, optic nerve tumors,
   neurofibromas of the cranial nerves, and
   meningiomas.

8. Young patients who present with seizures and no other neurological deficits may have an 87% 15-year survival if the tumor is a low grade astrocytoma.

PITFALLS:

1. Ten to fifteen percent of patients with low grade astrocytomas will go on to develop higher grade astrocytomas or glioblastomas in their clinical course.

2. A condition of widespread neoplastic transformation can occur throughout the cerebral hemispheres, brainstem, and cerebellum and is know as gliomatosis cerebri. This condition is usually seen in conjunction with neurofibromatosis or tuberous scleroses in the second and third decades of life. No mass effect may be detected on CT scan but diffusely narrowed ventricles, enlarged sulci, and an expanded brainstem and cerebellum may suggest the diagnosis.

3. Glioblastomas of the cerebellum, brainstem, and spinal cord are very rare. Lower grade astrocytomas are more common in the above locations.

4. Evidence of tumor recurrence in a patient treated with radiation therapy for a glioma must be distinguished from the latent effects of the radiation therapy itself, such as cyst formation, cerebritis, and radiation necrosis.

5. In mixed primary brain tumors, the clinical course of the patient is generally dictated by the most malignant portion of the tumor.

REFERENCES

1. Ciric I, Ammirati M, Vick N, et al: Supratentorial gliomas: surgical considerations and immediate post-operative results. Gross total resection versus partial resection. Neurosurgery 21(1):21-26, 1987.

2. Harsh GR, Levin VA, Gutin PH , et al: Re-operation for recurrent glioblastoma and anaplastic astrocytoma. Neurosurgery 21(5):615-621, 1987.

3. Jelsma R, Bury PC: The treatment of glioblastoma multiforme of the brain. J Neurosurg 27:388-400, 1967.

4. Kelly KA, Kirwood JM, Lapp DS: Glioblastoma multiforme: pathology, natural history and treatment. Cancer Treatment Rev 11:1-26, 1984.

5. Murovic J, Turowskik, Wilson CB, et al: Computerized tomography in the prognosis of malignant cerebral glioma. J Neurosurg 65(6): 799-806, 1986.

6. Saloman M: Survival in glioblastoma: historical perspective. Neurosurgery 7:435-439, 1980.

7. Saloman M, Kaplan RS, Ducker TB, Abdo H, Montgomery E: Effect of age and reoperation on survival in the combined modality treatment of malignant astrocytoma. Neurosurgery 10:454-463, 1982.

8. Shapiro WR: Treatment of neuroectodermal brain tumors. Ann Neurol 12:231-237, 1982.

9. Walker MD, Green SB, Byar DP, et al: Randomized comparison of radiotherapy and nitrosoureas for the treatment of malignant glioma after surgery. N Engl J Med 303:1323-1329, 1980.

SUDDEN HEADACHE AND ATAXIA IN AN ELDERLY HYPERTENSIVE WOMAN

CASE 14: This 74-year-old woman with known hypertension was well until she had an onset of a severe occipital headache with some neck stiffness. The patient had dizziness and difficulty walking with persistent falls to her right side. She was brought to the hospital after an episode of nausea, vomiting and confusion. In the emergency room, she was lethargic but arousable, had a right VI and VII nerve palsy, appendicular ataxia greater on her right than left, and a stiff neck. A computed tomography (CT) scan was obtained.

Clue:

CT scan

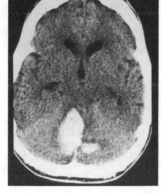

Figure 14.1

QUESTIONS:

1. What is the diagnosis?

2. Explain the symptoms of nausea, vomiting, lethargy, and stiff neck.

3. What are the possible etiologies?

4. What treatment would you recommend? Is this treatment always necessary?

5. If the patient rapidly deteriorated, what bedside maneuvers could be used to stabilize the patient prior to surgery?

ANSWERS:

1. The patient's history, symptoms, and CT scan are classic for an <u>acute cerebellar hematoma</u>. Although the clinical presentation of these pateints often points to posterior fossa pathology, the CT scan reveals the diagnosis without the need for a lumbar puncture which could precipitate herniation in this situation. The noncontrast CT reveals a large homogeneous mass in the right cerebellar hemisphere with shift of fourth ventricle from right to left and signs of early hydrocephalus with enlargement of the ventricles. Only intracerebellar blood can give this appearance on the CT scan.

2. The patient's symptoms are due to the direct effects of the hemorrhage on the cerebellum and the indirect effects of the pressure of the clot on the brain stem and ventricular system. Direct cerebellum dysfunction from the hemorrhage itself causes <u>ipsilateral appendicular ataxia</u> frequently presenting with the inability to walk or stand in these patients. Pressure on the right midpontine portion of the brain stem has resulted in the VIth and VIIth nerve palsies. The nausea/vomiting and stiff neck are caused by the <u>increased intracranial pressure</u> in the ventricular system as the mass effect of the hemorrhage obstructs the flow of cerebrospinal fluid (CSF) in the aqueduct and IVth ventricle. The stiff neck is usually not a sign of subarachnoid hemorrhage but instead one of partial cerebellar herniation (tonsilar portion) through the foramen magnum.

3. The majority of cerebellar hemorrhages in <u>hypertensive patients</u> can be traced to their hypertension. Other causes of intracerebellar bleeds include <u>trauma, vascular anomalies, [aneurysm and arteriovenous malformations (AVMs)], bleeding disorders, anticoagulation therapy, tumor bleeds, hemorrhagic infarction after cerebellar stroke, vasculitis, and amyloid angiopathy</u>.

4. A patient with a large intracerebellar hematoma and a deteriorating clinical course should be treated as <u>a neurosurgical emergency</u> and the clot should be evacuated as soon as possible. In situations in which the patient is clinically stable and the clot is less than 3 cm in diameter, an expectant course of treatment may be cautiously undertaken. The patient should be observed in an intensive care unit setting, steroids and mannitol may be required, and all necessary preparations for surgery should be made in case of any adverse change in the patient's neurological status.

5. A patient who rapidly deteriorates while under evaluation in the emergency room, in the intensive care unit, or awaiting surgery may be treated with <u>intubation, hyperventilation, steroids, mannitol, and a head gatch to 30—degrees to reduce acute intracranial pressure</u>. As the operating room is being readied for surgical evacuation of the clot, a ventricular drain should be placed at the bedside to treat acute hydrocephalus, if the above maneuvers have no effect.

PEARLS:

1. <u>Aneurysms are more frequent in the posterior fossa than AVMs</u>, however, most posterior fossa aneurysms present with subarachnoid hemorrhage as opposed to intraparencymal hemorrhages that occur with AVMs. AVMs in the posterior fossa are uncommon (10% of AVMs) but the possibility of a cerebellar hemorrhage resulting from an AVM should be considered in non-hypertensive patients under the age of 40 years. In such cases, angiography prior to surgery may be indicated.

2. <u>Cerebellar infarction or brain stem infarction</u> may have a similar clinical presentation as a cerebellar hematoma. An early CT scan can differentiate between these entities.

3. <u>The mental status is a strong prognostic indicator of outcome after surgery</u>. Those conscious or drowsy do well while those stuporous or comatose do poorly.

PITFALLS:

1. Postoperative deterioration in patients with
    cerebellar hematomas may be secondary to swelling
    in the posterior fossa resulting in acute
    hydrocephalus.

2. Do not confuse an _enhancing vermis_ on a contrast CT
    as a midline cerebellar hematoma. This is a normal
    finding on a contrast CT.

REFERENCES:

1. Auer LM: Indications for surgical treatment of
   cerebellar hemhorrage and infarction.   Acta
   Neurochir (Wein) 79(2-4):74-79, 1986.

2. Crowell RW, Ojemann RG: Cerebellar hemorrhage.   In
   Buchhert WA, Truex RC Jr, eds: Surgery of the
   posterior fossa. New York, Raven, 1979, pp 135-142.

3. Heiman TD, Satya-Murti S: Benign cerebellar
   hemorrhages. Ann Neurol 3:366-368, 1978.

4. Little JR, Tubman DE, Ethier R: Cerebellar
   hemorrhage in adults. Diagnosis by computerized
   tomography. J Neurosurg 48:575-579, 1978.

5. Macdonell RA, kalnis RM, Dunnan RG: Cerebellar
   infarction: natural history, prognosis, and
   pathology.   Stroke 18(5): 849-855, 1987.

6. Ott KH, Kase CS, Ojemann RG, Mohn JP: Cerebellar
   hemorrhage: diagnosis and treatment. A review of 56
   cases. Arch Neurol 31:160-167, 1974.

7. Taneda M: Primary cerebellar hemorrhage:
   quadrigeminal cistern obliteration on CT scans as a
   predictor of outcome.   J Neurosurg 67 (4):545-554,
   1987.

8. Weisberg LA: Acute cerebellar hemorrhage and CT
   evidence of tight posterior fossa.   Neurology 36
   (6):858-860, 1986.

ALTERED CONSCIOUSNESS AFTER HEAD INJURY

CASE 15: A 23-year-old man was playing baseball and while at bat was struck on the left side of his head by a wild pitch. He briefly appeared to be "dazed" according to his teammates but completed the game without incident. Approximately 1 hour later he appeared confused and then collapsed. On examination in the emergency room, he was noted to have a large bruise in the left temporal region of his head, an enlarged and poorly reactive left pupil, and a right hemiparesis. He was easily aroused but was disoriented and could not follow verbal commands.

Clue: CT SCAN OF HEAD

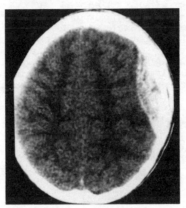

Figure 15.1

QUESTIONS:

1. Describe the likely x-ray findings in this patient and their significance.

2. What is the pathogenesis of this lesion?

3. How specific is this patient's clinical presentation for this condition?

4. What are the treatment and outcome for this condition?

85

ANSWERS:

1. A skull x-ray revealed the presence of a fracture in the left temporal bone. The noncontrast computed tomography (CT) scan demonstrates a hyperdense lenticular shaped mass between the skull and the brain causing a shift of the intracranial contents from left to right. This <u>combination of a temporal skull fracture and an underlying biconvex shaped hematoma on a CT scan in a head trauma patient is diagnostic of an epidural hematoma</u>. The presence of intracranial shift secondary to this hematoma signals impending cerebral herniation due to the displacement of the medial temporal lobe and uncus down through the tentorial notch which is immediately adjacent to these structures. The downward herniation of brain will cause compression of the ipsilateral IIIrd nerve and cerebral peduncle resulting in a dilated pupil on the side of the lesion and a hemiparesis contralateral to the hematoma. The hemiparesis is on the opposite side because the left cerebral peduncle carries motor fibers to the right side of the body that will eventually cross to the opposite side in the medulla which is well below the tentorial notch. This condition is a neurosurgical emergency which requires immediate attention.

2. Epidural hematomas are created in the potential space between the inner table of the skull and dura of the brain by a traumatic event that results in tearing of meningeal vessels and leakage of blood into this space. The most commonly involved meningeal vessel is <u>the middle meningeal artery</u> that enters the skull and joins the dura from the foramen spinosum at the skull base and travels up into the temporal fossa dura. This vessel gives branches to the frontal, parietal, and occipital dura in addition to the temporal area. In adults, <u>a skull fracture occurs in 90% of cases of epidural hematoma</u> but fractures are much less common in children as the skull is more compliant and the dura is less adherent to the inner table of the skull.

3. Epidural hematomas have become synonymous with the
    clinical description of a "lucid interval."   A
    lucid   interval   represents   the   period   of
    consciousness between the loss of consciousness at
    the moment of injury and the subsequent collapse
    into unconsciousness of the patient.

    Actually the lucid interval, as seen in this
    patient, is described in only approximately one
    third of patients with an epidural hematoma and is
    not pathognomonic of this condition as other types
    of   acute   central   nervous   trauma   injuries   may
    clinically express a lucid interval. Patients with
    an epidural hematoma may be conscious throughout
    their presentation, express a lucid interval at any
    point   during   their   presentation,   or   have   any
    combination of the above states of consciousness.

4. The   treatment   of   this   condition   is   immediate
    evacuation   of   the   hematoma   by   craniotomy   and
    coagulation of the bleeding sites on the dura.   In
    a rapidly deteriorating patient, an emergency burr
    hole may be placed on the side of the dilating
    pupil as a life-saving maneuver.   This does not
    represent definitive treatment, however, as it is
    usually not possible to remove the entire hematoma
    or identify dural bleeding points and should only
    be   intended   for   temporary   stabilization   of   the
    patient   prior   to   the   craniotomy.   Most   awake
    patients   can   be   stabilized   with   diuretics   and
    hyperventilation prior to surgery so that a CT scan
    delineating the complete extent of the injury may
    be obtained.   The outcome following treatment of an
    epidural hematoma is related to the age of the
    patient, presence of other associated intracranial
    injuries, the size and location of the hematoma,
    and most importantly the interval of time between
    the injury and surgery.   Almost all awake patients
    prior to surgery survive but comatose patients have
    up to a 40% mortality from this condition.   The
    most significant principle in the treatment of this
    condition is urgency.

PEARLS:

1. Epidural hematomas occur in only approximately 2% of all patients with craniocerebral trauma and is rare after the age of 60 years or before the age of 2 years.

2. Epidural hematomas may occur secondary to injury to meningeal veins, venous sinuses, or diploic veins. These patients may present with delayed or chronic epidural hematomas days after their injury.

3. Spontaneous cases of epidural hematomas may occur without trauma or a skull fracture and can be related to the presence of a dural arteriovenous malformation that has bled.

4. Posterior fossa epidural hematomas should be suspected in patients with skull fractures of the occipital bone, particularly those crossing the region of the traverse sinus. These hematomas are often unsuspected and may have a delayed presentation with signs of cerebellar compression or foramen magnum herniation. The mortality if unsuspected may reach 70%. They represent approximately 5% of all epidural hematomas.

PITFALLS:

1. Remember, epidural hematomas are not always temporal, not always secondary to middle meningeal artery injury, not always acute, not always associated with lucid intervals, and not always associated with a fracture skull.

2. Epidural hematomas on the cerebral vertex may be missed if high CT cuts are not included and thus a complete CT study to the top of the head is required in suspected patients.

3. Craniocerebral trauma patients frequently have injury to other organ systems that can be missed in an unconscious patient. Careful evaluation to preclude such emergencies as a cervical spine injury or a ruptured spleen should be part of the general approach to any unconscious trauma patient.

4. A false localizing hemiparesis on the side of the dilated pupil may be secondary to a <u>Kernohan's notch syndrome</u>. This condition can occur in an epidural hematoma and should not delay the treatment of this condition. This condition results from the compression of the opposite cerebral peduncle (on the side opposite of the hematoma) against the opposite tentorial edge as the brain stem is pushed to the opposite side from the herniating temporal lobe ipsilateral to the hematoma.

REFERENCES

1. Beller AJ, Peyer E: Extradural cerebellar hematoma: report of 3 cases with review of the literature. J Neurosurg 9:291-298, 1952.

2. Jamieson KG, Yellard JDN: Extradural hematoma: report of 167 cases. J Neurosurg 29:13-23, 1968.

3. Jawahar G, Natarajan M: Mortality in extradural hematoma. J Indian Med Assoc 85(8):235-237, 1987.

4. Lobato RD, Rivas JJ, Cordobes F, et al: Acute epidural hematoma: an analysis of factors influencing the outcome of patients undergoing surgery in coma. J Neurosurg 68(1):48-57, 1988.

5. Mendelow AD, Karmi MZ, Paul KS, Fullerg GAG, Gillingham FJ: Extradural hematoma: effect of delayed treatment. Br Med J 1:1240-1242, 1979.

6. Ponprosent C, Suwanwela C, Hongsaprablias C, Prichayudh P, O'Charoen S: Extradural hematoma: analysis of 138 cases. J Trauma 20:679-683, 1980.

7. Zimmerman RA, Bilanuik LT, Gennarelle T, Bruce D, Dolinskasc, Uzzell B: Cranial computed tomography in diagnosis and management of acute head trauma. AJR 131:27-34, 1978.

GUNSHOT WOUND TO THE HEAD

CASE 16: A 27-year-old man was shot in the right side of the head with a handgun during an assault. Initial examination in the emergency room revealed a stellate laceration of the scalp at the entrance site. There was no exit wound. Neurologically, he was lethargic, without speech or eye opening, but responded purposefully to pain (Glasgow Coma Scale = 7). Pupillary diameters were 5 mm on the right, 3 mm on the left; both were reactive, the right a bit sluggish. The remainder of the cranial nerves were intact. There was no gross asymmetry in limb strength. Reflexes were normal and active; plantar responses were flexor.

Subsequently the patient became increasingly obtunded. His right pupil dilated to 7 mm and did not react to light. He became hemiplegic on the right side with hyperreflexia and a right Babinski sign as well.

Plain anteroposterior (AP) and lateral skull x-rays revealed a comminuted fracture of the right temporal bone and showed the bullet and several smaller metal fragments restricted to the right side of midline. Computed tomography (CT) confirmed the comminuted fracture with many in-driven bony fragments and underlying contusion. The bullet and fragments penetrated the right frontal lobe. There was no ventricular or left hemisphere injury apparent. A large right subdural hematoma had also developed.

Neuroanatomical Clue:

The seemingly paradoxical development of hemiparesis ipsilateral to the IIIrd nerve palsy may be resolved by understanding the relationship of the cerebral peduncles to the tentorial edge which may result in a lesion known as Kernohan's notch (see diagram on next page).

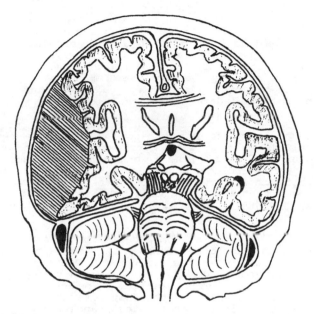

Figure 16.1

QUESTIONS:

1. Describe how the patient's presentation and course
   alert the surgeon to an expanding mass lesion on the
   right.

2. Explain the mechanisms of injury in gunshot wounds
   to the brain.

3. What are the goals of surgery?

4. What appropriate medical management should occur in
   the emergency room and perioperative period?

ANSWERS:

1. A decreased level of consciousness in any patient
    with head injury must always be presumed to be
    secondary to <u>elevated intracranial pressure</u>.
    Anisocoria, although present in many normal
    individuals, must also be considered significant in
    the head injured patient and is present in up to
    50% of patients with acute subdural hematomas.
    Often accompanied by sluggish reactivity, mild
    anisocoria may be present for hours before the
    pupil becomes fixed and dilated and further
    neurological deterioration occurs.

    Patients who are unresponsive or posturing
    immediately after a gunshot wound to the head and
    fail to improve with hyperventilation and osmotic
    diuresis have likely sustained diffuse brain
    injury, including the brain stem.   However,
    patients who are initially intact or purposeful and
    then deteriorate neurologically more commonly have
    <u>an expanding mass lesion</u> to account for their
    deterioration.

    The presence of hemiparesis ipsilateral to pupil
    dilation should not confuse the astute clinician to
    the location of the hematoma.   Pressure from the
    expanding hematoma pushes the brain stem laterally.
    The contralateral cerebral peduncle is then
    compressed against the opposite tentorial edge
    leading to ipsilateral motor changes.

2. The amount of brain injury sustained from a gunshot
    wound is <u>proportional to the amount of kinetic
    energy transferred from the bullet to the brain</u>.
    The transmitted energy in turn is dependent on the
    difference between the initial velocity, V_i, of the
    bullet at impact and the residual velocity, V_r,
    after leaving the brain, and the bullet mass is
    represented by the equation $E = 1/2 \ M \ (V_i{}^2 - V_r{}^2)$.
    As energy is proportional to the square of the
    velocity, this factor is more critical than the
    mass of the bullet in determining tissue
    disruption.   After the bullet enters the brain
    there is an immediate rise in intracranial pressure

secondary to shock waves that result in pressure
fluctuations as high as 1000 lb/in^2. This may
result in immediate herniation and death. A second
rise in intracranial pressure, up to 100 mm Hg,
occurs about 5 minutes after injury and is later
accompanied by a decrease in cerebral blood flow.
The bullet itself lacerates and crushes tissue
along its trajectory forming a <u>permanent</u> <u>cavity</u> the
diameter of which is slightly greater than the
diameter of the bullet. A <u>temporary cavity</u> is also
formed along the bullet path which only persists
for 10-20 ms. The size of the temporary cavity
increases with missile velocity and may reach
diameters 30 times the diameter of the missile.
Functional tissue disruption is proportional to the
area of the temporary cavity.

Hematomas and contusions may be produced
directly by the bullet along its path or indirectly
by displacement of the brain within the skull by
shock waves. Hematomas and contusions by the
latter mechanism often occur at a distance from the
bullet track. Subdural collections result from the
disruption of bridging veins or cortical vessels by
either mechanism.

3. The goals of surgery are:

   a) To remove hematomas and achieve
       hemostasis.
   b) To clean the bullet track removing
       debris, devitalized tissue, bone, and
       bullet fragments, where accessible
       <u>without increasing neurological
       deficit</u>, in order to minimize the
       risk of infection.
   c) Meticulous, watertight wound closure.
   d) To reduce the complications of
       elevated intracranial pressure
       postoperatively including the
       placement of intraventricular or
       subdural drains or pressure monitors
       where appropriate.

4. Control of elevated intracranial pressure (ICP) often demands immediate measures including <u>intubating and hyperventilating</u> the patient to lower the pCO_2 to 25-30 mm Hg and mannitol for osmotic diuresis. Steroids are also routinely administered although conclusive proof of their effectiveness is lacking.

    <u>Seizures following gunshot wounds</u> to the head may occur in up to 40% of patients. Therefore anticonvulsants should be given early. Phenytoin and phenobarbital are most commonly used acutely.

    <u>Adequate debridement and wound closure</u> are probably the critical factors in prevention of perioperative infection. Nevertheless prophylactic antibiotics are commonly used although this therapy also lacks support by controlled studies.

    Finally antacids and H_2-antagonists are often administered to prevent gastrointestinal hemorrhage.

PEARLS:

1. Overall mortality from gunshot wounds to the head has improved little despite recent advances in other areas of head injury. Mortality rates in recent civilian series range from 51 to 66%. <u>Almost 45% of civilian gunshot wounds to the head occur in suicide attempts</u>. Of the remaining 55% most result from assault.

    <u>The presenting neurological status of the patient is the best indicator of prognosis</u>. Patients who are awake and alert when first evaluated have a relatively low mortality ranging from 0 to 20%. Mortality among patients who are unresponsive at presentation approaches 90-100%. Recent studies have attempted to standardize data by comparing the correlation of the patient's score on the Glasgow Coma Scale (GCS) with mortality and outcome. The average GCS score for patients with good outcome was 9.5; those patients with poor outcome had an average GCS of 3.7. All patients with GCS of 13-15 survived whereas there were no survivors among patients with a GCS of 3. Other

important prognostic factors include bilateral hemispheric injury and ventricular injury, both of which are associated with poor outcome in 85-95% of cases. Patients with intracranial hematomas also do worse.

2. Gunshot wounds to the head in military situations differ from civilian injuries in several ways. First <u>military wounds often are inflicted by rifles with high muzzle velocities</u>, in excess of 750 m/s, and as a result have a higher mortality. Handguns with low muzzle velocities (<250 m/s) are more common in civilian situations resulting in lower mortality and less extensive injury to the scalp and skull. Handgun bullets more commonly fail to exit the skull and may ricochet back into the brain along a different path. Finally military wounds are dirtier and more destructive than civilian ones and extensive debridement, even reoperation for missed fragments of bone and metal, is more critical in the prevention of infection.

3. <u>The gunshot victim who presents in coma, unresponsive to pain, and with fixed and dilated pupils (GCS = 3) rarely survives</u> with or without surgery and is not generally considered an operative candidate. Patients with a higher level of consciousness initially who subsequently deteriorate often have an operative lesion such as an expanding hematoma and may benefit from surgery.

PITFALLS:

1. <u>Traumatic aneurysms and arteriovenous fistulas</u> are commonly associated with inferior cranial wounds. These may be missed initially since CT scanning has replaced arteriography as the procedure of choice following gunshot wounds to the head. Therefore, angiography should be considered when gunshot wounds involve this location.

2. <u>Dural sinuses</u>, more commonly injured in military than civilian wounds, may be the source of profuse bleeding. Ligation of the precoronal sagittal sinus or nondominant transverse sinus can usually be done safely. Obstruction of other sinuses, however, may be fatal and necessitate repair.

REFERENCES

1. Clark WC, Muhlbauer MS, Watridge CB, Ray MW: Analysis of 76 civilian craniocerebral gunshot wounds. J Neurosurg 65:9-14, 1986.

2. Cooper PR: Gunshot wounds of the brain. In Cooper PR, ed. Head injury. Baltimore, Williams & Wilkins, 1982, pp 257-274.

3. Hogan RE: Early complications following penetrating wounds of the brain. J Neurosurg 34:134-141, 1971.

4. Hammon WM: Analysis of 2,187 consecutive penetrating wounds to the brain from Vietnam. J Neurosurg 34: 127-131, 1971.

5. Hubschmann O, Shapiro K, Baden M, Schulman K: Craniocerebral gunshot injuries in civilian practice-prognostic criteria and surgical management: experience with 82 cases. J Trauma 19:6-12, 1979.

6. Kirkpatrick JB, Dimaio V: Civilian gunshot wounds of the brain. J Neurosurg 49:185-198, 1978.

7. Kaufman HH, Makela ME, Lee KF, Haid RW, Gildenberg PL: Gunshot wounds to the head: a perspective. Neurosurgery 18:689-695, 1986.

8. Harsh GR III, Harsh GR IV,: Penetrating wounds of the head. In Wilkins RH, Rengachary SS, eds. Neurosurgery. Baltimore, Williams & Wilkins 1985, pp 1670-1678.

HEADACHE AND VISUAL LOSS

CASE 17:   The patient was a 40-year-old man who presented with occasional headaches and difficulty reading. On physical examination he was found to have a bitemporal visual field cut, more severe in the lower quadrant. The remainder of the neurological exam was within normal limits. Computed tomography (CT) scan revealed a cystic mass in the suprasellar region with some calcification. Pre-operative endocrinological testing revealed no abnormalities. Pathology was consistent with craniopharyngioma.

Neuroanatomical Clue:

The nature of the visual field loss gives information as to the position and the possible nature of the mass.   The fibers from the superior nasal portion of the retina (which monitor the inferior temporal visual field) cross in the posterior portion of the optic chiasm.   Craniopharyngiomas frequently arise posterior to the chiasm; thus, the inferior temporal visual fields are the first to be affected by the pressure of the growing tumor.   In contrast, a pituitary adenoma growing out of the sella will frequently compress the anterior aspect of chiasm first.   In this case the fibers affected initially are those serving the superior temporal visual fields.

QUESTIONS:

1. From what embryological structure are craniopharyngiomas thought to arise?

2. What is the differential diagnosis for a mass in the suprasellar region?

3. What findings on various neuroradiological procedures help to confirm the diagnosis?

4. What is the operative approach to this tumor?

5. What forms of adjunctive therapy may aid in the management of the tumor?

6. How may this presentation differ in the pediatric age group?

ANSWERS:

1. The pituitary gland develops from two distinct
    structures.   In the third week of gestation, an
    evagination of the stomodeum appears just in front
    of the buccopharyngeal membrane.   This structure,
    known as Rathke's pouch, grows dorsally to meet a
    downward extension of the diencephalon - the
    infundibulum.   Rathke's pouch goes on to form the
    anterior   lobe   of   the   pituitary,   while   the
    infundibulum becomes the stalk and the posterior
    lobe. Craniopharyngiomas are thought to arise from
    remnants of Rathke's pouch and thus may be found at
    any location along the path of migration from the
    pharynx to the suprasellar region. The most common
    location is anterior to the stalk of the pituitary,
    with dense adhesion to this structure.

2. The differential diagnosis of a suprasellar mass
    includes meningioma, hypothalamic glioma, pituitary
    adenoma,   teratoma,   aneurysm,   hamartoma,
    craniopharyngioma,   metastasis,   chordoma,   bony
    tumors and sinus mucoceles.

3. Computed tomographic (CT) scan currently provides
    the best diagnostic information. Craniopharyngiomas
    tend to be bulky with a prominent cystic component
    although they occasionally are solid.   They
    frequently contain calcifications both centrally
    and at the rim.   They enhance with contrast
    administration.

        Plain skull films may reveal calcifications in
    the suprasellar region.   Ballooning of the sella
    may be seen if the tumor has a sellar extension.

        Angiography   is   helpful   preoperatively   to
    determine the relationship of the tumor to the
    arteries of the circle of Willis, especially the
    internal carotid arteries.

        Magnetic   resonance   imaging   provides   both
    excellent anatomical detail and the capability of
    providing sagittal and coronal images to better
    visualize the extent of the lesion.

4. The operative approach to the lesion is dependent on the exact extent of the lesion. From the characteristic origin on the anterior aspect of the pituitary stalk, the tumor may grow upward toward the third ventricle and hypothalamus, forward toward the chiasm and anterior fossa, downward towards the sella, or backward toward the posterior fossa. The standard approach is via a frontal craniotomy, underneath the frontal lobes and through the spaces between the carotid artery and optic nerve. It is sometimes necessary to approach the sellar portion (if it is present) through a separate, transsphenoidal approach. It is frequently possible to drain the cyst, making the remainder of the dissection easier.

A controversy exists regarding the need for complete removal versus conservative resection. These tumors have a dense glial reaction surrounding them, and are frequently closely adherent to surrounding structures, including the hypothalamus, the pituitary stalk, the carotid arteries, and the optic nerves. A radical resection places all of these structures at risk, but some surgeons feel this is the only way to achieve an adequate success rate in terms of survival and recurrence.

If the cerebrospinal fluid (CSF) pathways are compromised, a shunting procedure may be necessary prior to attempting resection of the tumor.

5. Radiation is the primary adjunctive therapy. This may be delivered as conventional, external brain radiation or by the injection of various radioactive compounds into the cystic portion of the tumor. Some authors report good response to radiation therapy and advocate conservative surgical procedures combined with radiation therapy. Others are less in favor of radiation in this region, especially in children, because of the chronic sequelae of radiation on the endocrine and cognitive functions.

For recurrent tumors, radiation is a mainstay of therapy, although reoperation is becoming more frequent. For nonresectable tumors where the cystic component leads to pressure and neurological deficits, a catheter may be placed into the cystic portion for decompression and palliation of symptoms.

6. Adult patients typically present with visual complaints, and a high percentage will have visual deficits on examination. A large percentage will have endocrine dysfunction as well.

    Children are less sensitive to visual impairment, and may tolerate a large degree of visual loss. For this reason, tumors in this group may grow to a large size and obstruct the CSF pathways. The child then presents with increased intracranial pressure: headache, nausea, vomiting, and papilledema.

PEARLS:

1. Ten to fifteen percent of adults with craniopharyngiomas may present with psychosis or disturbance in mentation, frequently in association with hydrocephalus.

2. Craniopharyngiomas represent approximately 3% of brain tumors. Fifty percent present before 20, and they represent 9% of the brain tumors in the pediatric age group.

3. Although craniopharyngiomas are believed to be derived from remnants of Rathke's pouch, they are histologically distinct from the benign Rathke's pouch cyst.

PITFALLS:

1. Because of adherence to suprasellar structures, safe removal via the transsphenoidal approach is difficult except in the unusual case of an intrasellar craniopharyngioma.

2. The blood supply to the inferior hypothalamus is derived from small branches of the posterior communicating artery which can be compromised during resection of a craniopharyngioma.

3. The origin and adherence of craniopharyngioma at
    the pituitary stalk make <u>postoperative endocrine
    deficits likely</u>.   Diabetes insipidus is frequent,
    and screening for all aspects of pituitary function
    is mandatory to determine the optimal replacement
    required.

REFERENCES

1. Carmel PW: Craniopharyngiomas.   In Neurosurgery,
   Wilkins RH, Rengarchary SS, eds. New York, McGraw-
   Hill, 1985, pp 905-915.

2. Daniels DL: Sellar and juxtasellar region.   In
   Cranial computed tomography. Williams AL, Haughton
   VM, eds. St. Louis, CV Mosby, 1985, p 444.

3. Kemps LG: Operative neurosurgery, Volume 1.   N e w
   York, Springer-Verlag, 1968, pp 90-94.

4. Kornblith PL, Walker MD, Cassidy JR: Neurologic
   Oncology. JJ Trippincott Co., 1987, pp 181-193.

5. Langman J: Medical embryology. Baltimore, Williams
   & Wilkins, 1901, p 341.

6. Patten J: Neurological differential diagnosis.
   New York, Springer Verlag, 1982, pp 11-26.

7. Sweet   WH: Craniopharyngiomas.   In   Operative
   neurosurgical techniques, Vol 1. Schmidek HH, Sweet
   WH, eds. New York, Grune-Stratton, 1982, pp 291.

ACUTE ONSET OF SEVERE HEADACHE WITH ASSOCIATED NAUSEA, VOMITING, AND STIFF NECK

<u>CASE 18</u>: A 43-year-old man noted the acute onset of severe occipital headache during strenuous exercise. Shortly after the appearance of the headache, the patient experienced several episodes of nausea and vomiting. There was no loss of consciousness.

Initial evaluation in the emergency room revealed the patient to be in moderate distress from "the worst headache of my life." Neurological exam was normal.

Lumbar puncture revealed grossly bloody cerebrospinal fluid with an opening pressure of 300 mm water. A computed tomography (CT) scan was reported as normal. The patient was placed on strict bed rest with the presumptive diagnosis of aneurysmal subarachnoid hemorrhage. On hospital day 4, a cerebral angiogram was performed which revealed a 1 cm aneurysm at the basilar bifurcation.

On day 7, his neurological condition was unchanged from admission. The patient underwent a frontotemporal craniotomy with clipping of the basilar artery aneurysm. Postoperatively, the patient did well except for a complete right oculomotor nerve palsy. Cerebral angiography, performed 1 week postoperatively, showed complete obliteration of the aneurysm. Return of third nerve function began soon after surgery with complete recovery by 3 months postoperatively.

CLUE: Preoperative cerebral angiogram.

Figure 18.1

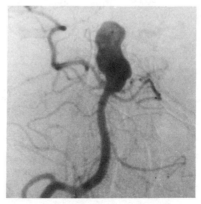

QUESTIONS:

1. The vascular system of the brain is traditionally divided into anterior and posterior circulations. Describe these two circulations.

2. What percentage of intracranial aneurysms arise from the vertebrobasilar system? Describe the most common locations of ancurysms of the posterior circulation.

3. What are the clinical syndromes produced by aneurysms arising from the basilar artery?

4. What is the most effective treatment of basilar artery aneurysms?

ANSWERS:

1. The anterior circulation, or carotid circulation, consists of all cerebral vasculature derived from both carotid arteries. Included in this system are the <u>anterior and middle cerebral arteries</u> which supply the anterior three-fourths of the cerebral hemispheres. Small perforating vessels arising from proximal segments of the internal carotid, anterior cerebral, and middle cerebral arteries supply important deep structures of the brain including the internal capsule, basal ganglia, and the anterior portions of the diencephalon.

    The <u>posterior circulation, or vertebrobasilar system</u>, consists of all vessels arising from the vertebral and basilar arteries. The basilar artery is a single artery formed by the fusion of both vertebral arteries, which occurs at the pontomedullary junction. The posterior circulation supplies the cerebellum, posterior diencephalon, as well as the entire midbrain, pons, and medulla. The posterior one fourth of the cerebral hemispheres and much of the inferior surface of the cerebral cortex are supplied by the vertebrobasilar system via the posterior cerebral arteries.

    <u>Paired posterior communicating arteries unite the anterior and posterior circulations</u>. A single anterior communicating artery connects the anterior cerebral arteries completing an arterial network at the base of the brain known as the **circle of Willis**. Variation in this network, due to hypoplasia of one or more of these communicating arteries, is common so that only a minority of the general population possess a truly competent circle of Willis. Anomalies of this circle are particularly common in patients with cerebral aneurysms and are probably causally related.

2. <u>The majority of intracranial aneurysms involve the anterior circulation</u>. Only **5 TO 10%** of all intracranial aneurysms arise from the vertebrobasilar system. The most common location of vertebrobasilar aneurysms is at the <u>basilar bifurcation</u>. The next most common locations are the

basilar trunk and the vertebral artery at the
origin of the posterior inferior cerebellar artery.

3. The most common clinical presentation of basilar
    artery aneurysm is <u>subarachnoid hemorrhage</u> produced
    by rupture of the aneurysm. The syndrome of
    subarachnoid hemorrhage is classically represented
    in the case report. Less commonly, the aneurysm may
    act as a mass lesion producing focal neurological
    deficits from compression of adjacent neural
    structures, particularly the cerebral peduncles and
    oculomotor nerves. Giant basilar aneurysms may
    compress the aqueduct of Sylvius producing a non-
    communicating hydrocephalus. Focal neurological
    deficits may also be produced by emboli arising
    from the thrombus within the aneurysm.

4. <u>Surgical obliteration of the aneurysm by applying a
    clip across the aneurysm neck</u> is the preferred
    method of treatment. If there is no definable neck,
    then hunterian ligation of the aneurysm by
    occlusion of the basilar artery above the origin of
    the superior cerebellar arteries may be possible.
    This maneuver depends on adequate collateral
    circulation from both posterior communicating
    arteries which may be determined during angiography
    or at surgery. If clipping or isolation of the
    aneurysm is not possible, then wrapping of the
    aneurysm with muslin may reduce, but does not
    eliminate, the risk of future rupture of the
    aneurysm.

PEARLS:

1. <u>The most common cause of spontaneous subarachnoid
    hemorrhage in the adult population is rupture of an
    intracranial aneurysm.</u> Under the age of 20 years
    vascular anomalies, particulary arteriovenous
    malformations, are the most common cause of
    spontaneous subarachnoid hemorrhage. Rarer causes
    of subarachnoid hemorrhage include blood
    dyscrasias, arteritis, Moya Moya disease, and
    tumors.

2. About 20% of patients with intracranial aneurysm
    have <u>multiple aneurysms</u>. Multiple aneurysms are
    more common in women.

3. Complete 4 vessel angiography is essential in the evaluation of patients suspected of harboring an intracranial aneurysm. This allows the identification of additional aneurysms as well as defining the extent of vasospasm and identifying variations of the patient's intracranial vascular system which could affect treatment.

PITFALLS:

1. Headache is a rather common presenting symptom in patients seeking medical attention. Although only a small percentage of these patients will have a subarachnoid hemorrhage (SAH) as a cause of their headache, the importance of prompt recognition of SAH and early treatment of aneurysms cannot be overstressed. Each year a significant percentage of patients with aneurysmal SAH have a delay in diagnosis even though they presented for medical attention shortly after their hemorrhage. Unnecessary delays in the diagnosis of SAH put the patient at increased risk for rerupture and vasospasm.

REFERENCES

1. Drake CG: The treatment of aneurysms of the posterior circulations. Clin Neurosurg 26:96-144, 1979.

2. Logue V: Posterior fossa aneurysms. Clin Neurosurg 11:183-219, 1964.

3. Solomon RA, Fink ME: Current strategies for management of aneurysmal subarachnoid hemorrhage. Arch Neurol 44:769-774, 1987.

4. Sugita K, Kobayashi S, Takemae T, et al: Aneurysms of the basilar artery trunk. J Neurosurg 66:500-505, 1987.

5. Troupp H: The natural history of aneurysms of the basilar bifurcation. Acta Neurol Scand 47:350-356, 1971.

HOMONYMOUS HEMIANOPSIA WITH RECURRENT HEADACHE AND WEAKNESS

CASE 19:   This 30-year-old right-handed woman in excellent health until 4 years prior to evaluation when she suddenly fell with mild right-sided weakness that resolved gradually over several days.   She had a similar episode 2 years ago with the addition of right-sided visual loss and severe headache that resolved over several hours.   A third episode of severe headache, nausea, right-sided weakness, and visual difficulties occurred immediately prior to her current evaluation; however, the right visual deficit did not resolve.   Neurological examination revealed the presence of a right homonymous hemianopsia.   The remainder of the examination was entirely normal. A computed tomography (CT)scan and angiogram were performed.

Clue: CT scan and angiogram

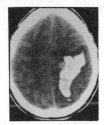   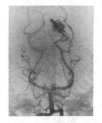

Figure 19.1 (left)   Figure 19.1 (right)

QUESTIONS:

1. Describe the CT findings in this case and what is the diagnosis?

2. What types of vascular malformations are found in the central nervous system (CNS), how are they defined pathologically, and what is their incidence?

3. What is the natural history of this lesion?

4. What treatments are available for this condition?

5. What factors are important when considering surgery in these patients and would you recommend surgery in this patient?

107

ANSWERS:

1.   The CT scan reveals the presence of a left
     occipital lobe hemorrhage (with serpiginous vessels
     on the contrast scan surrounding the region of the
     hemorrhage).   This pattern is suggestive of an
     arteriovenous   malformation   (AVM)   which   was
     confirmed by angiography.   The angiogram reveals
     the presence of a large dilated posterior cerebral
     vessel that is the primary arterial input to this
     malformation and several draining veins to the
     sagittal sinus.   The angiogram is diagnostic for
     AVM and is critical in determining the location of
     the major arterial inputs and venous drainage of
     these lesions.   Special techniques such as
     magnification   angiography   and   stereoscopic
     angiography are useful adjuncts to the surgeon in
     understanding the fine detail and 3 dimensional
     configuration of AVMs.

2.   Most pathologists subdivide the vascular
     malformations of the brain into 4 groups, each
     having its own pathology, natural history, and
     clinical management.   In order of descending
     frequency these lesions are: venous malformations,
     telangiectases, arteriovenous malformations, and
     cavernous malformations, with only the latter 2
     lesions   requiring   neurosurgical   intervention.
     Venous malformations are anomalous veins separated
     by normal brain tissue usually located in the deep
     white matter with a radial configuration on
     angiography in the venous phase.   They do not have
     arterial inputs and rarely result in clinical
     symptoms such as hemorrhage or thrombosis.
     Surgical resection may result in venous infarction
     of the surrounding brain and is therefore rarely
     indicated.

         Telangiectases are clusters of small capillary-
     like vessels found most frequently in the pons.
     They do not visualize on CTs or angiograms and are
     generally found on postmortem examinations of the
     brain.

Cavernous malformations consist of a cluster of
tightly packed sinusoidal type vessels without
intervening brain tissue.   Grossly they appear
mulberry like and are frequently calcified.   The
lesions frequently occur in the subcortical white
matter of the frontal or temporal lobes but may be
found in any location in the CNS including the
spinal cord and brain stem.   These malformations
can and do hemorrhage and rarely visually on
angiograms because of their meager arterial input.
Magnetic resonance imaging (MRI) and CT are useful
in suggesting the diagnosis as calcium density,
flowing blood, and hemorrhage can be detected in
the studies.   Surgical excision is required both
for diagnosis and for the prevention of additional
hemorrhages.

AVMs are collections of abnormal arteries and
veins in communication with one another without an
intervening capillary bed that frequently contain
neurnal parenchyma within their boundaries.   The
vessels are quite abnormal pathologically and may
be thickened, hylinized, or contain calcium.   Blood
flow through these malformations is quite high and
this abnormal flow may divert or "steal" blood
supply from surrounding brain areas resulting in
neurological deficits.   Frequent evidence at the
time of surgery of clinically silent hemorrhage is
found in AVMs and the surrounding brain may be
gliotic or calcified.   Surgical and radiological
interventions are frequently necessary to prevent
rebleeding from these lesions.

3. The natural history of AVMs is incompletely known
but the clinical presentation and course are
greatly influenced by the age of the patient.   AVMs
are considered congenital lesions although they
infrequently present the first decade of life.
When they do occur early in life, heart failure,
hydrocephalus, and seizures are the most common
modes of presentation.   Symptomatic AVMs generally
occur in the third to the fourth decades with the
majority of patients suffering headaches,
hemorrhages, seizures, or neurological deficits as
a result of the presence of the AVM.   The most

serious risk, that of hemorrhage, occurs at the rate of 2 to 3% per year in this age group. Those patients that have a hemorrhage incur a 10% mortality from this event in addition to an increased risk of rehemorrhage of 6% in the first year after the initial bleed. After this period of time, it is estimated that one-third of the patients will remain well, 28% will have mild deficits, 29% will be disabled, and 10% will die as a result of their AVM. In a symptomatic patient in the middle years of life a mortality rate of 1-2% per year and a morbidity rate of 3-4% per year can be expected. During the fifth decade of life and beyond, the risk of hemorrhage and morbidity decreases compared to the middle decades and may represent that an equilibrium between the AVM and the surrounding brain has been reached in this older age group.

4. Treatments available for the management of AVMs include the following: a) surgical resection b) intravascular embolization with silastic pellets, balloons, or bucrylate c) a combination of the above two modalities d) proton beam irradiation e) conservative therapy without any of the above interventions.

5. Factors important in the surgical decision making process for an AVM include the age of the patient, a clinical presentation with a hemorrhage, the accessibility of the lesion surgically, and the degree of difficulty anticipated in resecting the lesion. In this particular patient, we have a young patient presenting with a hemorrhage secondary to a relatively small AVM in an accessible location. Because of the increased risk of rebleeding in this age group and the anticipation of a complete resection, surgery is clearly indicated. Had this lesion been larger or in a more eloquent region of the brain, a staged procedure consisting of embolization first and surgery later may have been indicated.

PEARLS:

1. Approximately 6% of AVMs are multiple and 8% are associated with aneurysms, usually located on the feeding vessels to the AVM.

2. Angiographically occult or "cryptic" AVMs may mimic the symptoms of a primary (or metastatic) brain tumor or hypertensive hemorrhage. Only surgery can establish the diagnosis as these infrequent lesions do no visualize as AVMs on angiograms and are usually discovered to represent cavenous malformation at surgery.

3. The vein of Galen malformation presents in neonates with a cranial bruit, hydrocephalus, and cardiomegaly. This high flow arteriovenous fistula can result in heart failure if not treated promptly.

4. Vasospasm is rare in hemorrhage from AVMs.

5. AVMs are frequently pyramidal in shape with the base on the cortex and the apex pointing toward the ventricle.

6. Ninety percent of AVMs are supratentorial and 10% are infratentorial.

7. Cranial bruit is highly suggestive of an underlying malformation but is only infrequently heard.

8. The presence of a cutaneous vascular skin lesion may point to an underlying cerebral vascular anomaly such as in the Sturge-Weber syndrome. In this condition a "port wine" stain is found in the cutaneous distribution of the trigeminal nerve and is associated with an underlying cortical malformation that results in hemiparesis, frequent seizures, and occasional mental retardation.

PITFALLS:

1. Nine percent of subarachnoid hemorrhage and 1% of strokes are associated with cerebral AVMs.

2. The presence of single or multiple subarachnoid hemorrhage with negative cerebral angiography may imply the existence of a spinal cord AVM. These lesions are one-tenth as common as cerebral AVMs and may occur either within the cord substance itself or on the outside of the cord.

3. Autoregulation of the cerebral vascular system around an AVM may be impaired after the resection of an AVM. This can lead to an inability of the cerebral vessels to cope with the increased flow in the brain surrounding the resected AVM and may result in hemorrhage or increased intracranial pressure postoperatively.

4. Venous malformations and venous varix (dilated vein) rarely present as symptomatic lesions and surgical resection is usually complicated by venous infarction.

5. Cerebellar hemorrhages in patients under 40 years of age are usually secondary to AVMs or tumor hemorrhages.

6. Cranial bruits occasionally are due to AVMs of the underlying dura and not the cortex. Dural malformations are rare and may also present with hemorrhage and very rarely dementia. The treatment is surgical excision of the dura, embolization, or observation depending upon the size, location, and symptoms of the dural malformation.

REFERENCES

1. Michelsen WJ: Natural history and pathophysiology of arteriovenous malformations. Neurosurgery 26:307, 1979.

2. Spetzler RF, Wilson CB, Weinstein P, et al: Normal perfusion pressure breakthrough theory. Neurosurgery 25:651, 1978.

3. Stein BM, Wolpert SM: Arteriovenous malformations of the brain.I: Current concepts and treatment. Arch Neurol 37:1, 1980.

PROGRESSIVE OBTUNDATION AFTER HEAD TRAUMA

CASE 20: A 43-year-old man was brought into the emergency room after having been found confused and speaking incoherently on a park bench. No further history was available.

In the emergency room, he became more obtunded, with no spontaneous speech and no response to verbal commands. The left parietal scalp had a large area of subcutaneous swelling and contusion from probable blunt trauma. His left pupil was fixed and dilated. His right pupil was fully reactive and corneal reflexes were intact. There was spontaneous movement in all of his extremities, although with greater frequency on his right side. Respirations were 30 per minute with some irregularity.

QUESTIONS:

1. What should be the initial management of this patient?

2. What is the neuroradiological procedure of choice to establish the cause of his neurological deficits?

Clue: Computed tomography (CT) Scan

Figure 20.1

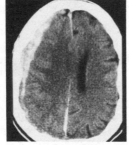

3. What is the pathophysiology demonstrated on the CT scan?

4. What is the management of this condition?

5. What is the prognosis with this type of injury?

ANSWERS:

1. From rapid evaluation of this clinical situation,
    it is likely that this patient has recently had
    significant head trauma resulting in progressive
    neurological dysfunction. As with any type of
    trauma, the same basic rules of <u>rapid airway
    control and circulatory support</u> apply. The patient
    should be intubated to gain control of his
    respirations and hyperventilated to lower his
    intracranial pressure. These measures should be
    carried out before any diagnostic studies.

2. When a patient presents with a deteriorating
    clinical course, there is no time for extensive,
    time-consuming radiological studies which may cause
    delays in treatment. The preferred radiological
    procedure is a CT scan. <u>A CT scan will adequately
    visualize the entire intracranial contents along
    with associated skull fractures, hematomas,
    contusions and edema</u>. A skull x-ray may be helpful
    if a skull fracture is present, however, the x-rays
    are often of poor quality when taken on a portable
    machine in the emergency room. More importantly, a
    skull x-ray is not a reliable predictor of the site
    of an intracranial contusion or hematoma and is
    unlikely to alter treatment plans if an adequate CT
    scan can be completed.

3. The patient has <u>a subdural hematoma</u>. This is
    usually caused by blunt trauma to the head leading
    to rupture of cortical vessels or tearing of
    cortical bridging veins. The blood in the subdural
    space spreads out over the convexity of the brain
    and acts as an evolving intracranial mass to
    produce neurological dysfunction. The impact
    producing this injury is usually of sufficient
    severity to cause direct injury to underlying brain
    parenchyma. Direct injury to the brain contributes
    to the generally poor prognosis associated with
    acute subdural hematoma.

4. A patient with a progressive neurological
    <u>deterioration secondary to subdural hematoma
    constitutes a neurosurgical emergency</u> warranting
    the prompt evacuation of the clot. While surgical

preparations are being made, immediate management consists of measures to lower intracranial pressure, specifically hyperventilation and intravenous mannitol. The efficacy of large dose steroids is unproven and controversial.

Surgical treatment consists of a wide exposure of the brain with a craniotomy centered over the maximal thickness of the hematoma. The dura is incised and the hematoma is carefully evacuated. Only frankly devitalized brain is resected and hemostasis is obtained. The clot is usually stiff in consistency rendering a burr hole inadequate for satisfactory evacuation. During the closure of the craniotomy, a drain is left in the subdural space and brought out through a separate stab wound to allow for more drainage and prevent further accumulation of blood. Finally, a ventricular drain or subarachnoid bolt is placed to monitor postoperative intracranial pressure.

5. Patients with subdural hematomas generally have an unsatisfying outcome, probably related to the associated cortical brain contusion that invariably accompanies the trauma. The mortality rate is approximately 35 to 50% and there is rarely a return to normal function. Some particularly poor prognostic factors are advanced age, unconsciousness at the time of injury, and delay in treatment.

PEARLS:

1. Patients should receive prophylactic anticonvulsants for at least 1 year. Seizures occur in one third of patients following cortical injury.

2. The mass effect from a subdural hematoma will usually cause a shift of the ventricles. This shift is easily visualized on CT scan, which is helpful in making the diagnosis when the hematoma is small. However, 15 to 20% of hematomas, are bilateral, which leads to ventricular compression without any noticeable shift from the midline.

PITFALLS:

1.   Diagnostic and therapeutic measures must proceed as
     rapidly as possible in patients with head trauma.
     Studies have shown that the mortality rate
     decreases from 90 to 30% in patients with acute
     subdural hematomas when surgery is performed within
     4 hours after injury.

2.   A high index of suspicion for <u>associated cervical
     fracture</u> must be maintained when treating patients
     with significant head trauma. When the
     circumstances surrounding a patient's head injury
     are unclear, a cervical collar should be placed
     until adequate cervical spine x-rays are obtained.

3.   Postoperatively up to 50% of patients with acute
     subdural hematomas experience further deterioration
     due to increased intracranial pressure. When
     deterioration occurs, a CT scan may be necessary to
     distinguish <u>cerebral edema</u> (requiring medical
     management) from delayed or residual hematoma
     (requiring surgical treatment).

4.   As with epidural hematomas, many patients with
     subdural hematoma experience a <u>"lucid interval"</u>
     immediately following trauma. Patients with
     significant head trauma must be examined frequently
     for signs of deterioration which may occur with
     progressive accumulation of a hematoma.

5.   The neurological exam may be misleading in terms of
     localizing the site of a subdural hematoma. In
     some instances hemiparesis occurs ipsilateral to
     the hematoma if <u>the opposite cerebral peduncle is
     compressed against the tentorial edge (Kernohan's
     notch)</u>. Less common is contralateral pupillary
     dilatation secondary to oculomotor nerve
     compression against the tentorium or direct injury
     to the orbit. Pupillary abnormalities may also
     occur with brain stem injury.

REFERENCES

1. Bender MB, Christoff N: Nonsurgical treatment of subdural hematomas. Arch Neurol 31:73-79, 1974.

2. Braun J, Borovich B, Guilburd JN, et al: Acute subdural hematoma mimicking epidural hematoma on CT. AJNR 8(1):171-173, 1987.

3. Cooper PR: Traumatic intracranial hematomas, in Wilkins RH, Rengachary SS, eds: Neurosurgery. McGraw-Hill Co., New York, 1985, pp 1657-1666.

4. Cooper PR, Rovit RL, Ransohoff J: Hemicraniectomy in the treatment of acute subdural hematoma: a reappraisal. Surg Neurol 5:25-28, 1976.

5. Fell DA, Fitzgerald S, Moiel RH, Caram P: Acute subdural hematomas: review of 144 cases. J Neurosurg 42:37-42, 1975.

6. Rockswold GL, Leonard PR, Nagib MG: Analysis of management in 33 closed head injury patients who "talked and deteriorated." Neurosurgery 21 (1):51-55, 1987.

7. Seelig JM, Becker DP, Miller JD, et al: Traumatic acute subdural hematoma. N Engl J Med 304:1511-1518, 1981.

8. Stone JL, Rifai MHS, Sugar O, et al: Subdural hematomas: I. Acute subdural hematoma: progress in definition, clinical pathology, and therapy. Surg Neurol 19:216-231, 1983.

9. Tokoro K, Nakajima F, Yamataki A: Acute spontaneous subdural hematoma of arterial origin. Surg Neurol 29(2):159-163, 1988.

HEADACHE AND IMPAIRED UPGAZE

CASE 21:   A 29-year-old man presented with a 1-month
history of recurrent headaches. Headaches were worse
in the morning, and on the day prior to admission his
headache was constant and associated with nausea and
vomiting.   His family had noticed some recent subtle
changes in his personality including apathy and
forgetfulness.

On examination he was slightly agitated and had
difficulty concentrating. His visual acuity and visual
fields were normal, but fundoscopic examination
revealed bilateral papilledema.   Ocular testing
revealed impaired convergence and upgaze with
retraction nystagmus.   Pupils were sluggishly reactive
to light but briskly reactive to accommodation.   There
was mild anisocoria.   Other cranial nerves were intact.
Motor and sensory testing was unremarkable but there
was mild gait ataxia on attempted tandem walking.

Clue:

The following magnetic resonance imaging (MRI) scan
was obtained: (Figure 21.1)

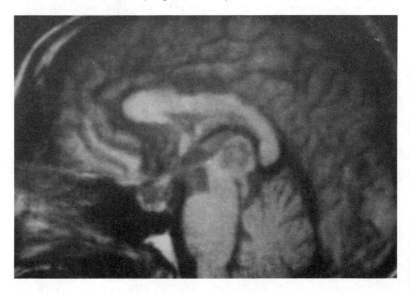

QUESTIONS:

1. Describe the anatomical location of this patient's lesion in terms of his symptoms and MRI scan.

2. What types of tumors are found in this location?

3. What is involved in the preoperative workup of this patient?

4. What is the role of surgery in these tumors?

5. What is the postoperative management of patients with unresectable tumors?

6. How is the hydrocephalus managed?

ANSWERS:

1.   The patient has a <u>tumor of the pineal region</u>. His symptoms are due to two separate processes: <u>hydrocephalus and midbrain compression</u>. The tumor has caused occlusion of the aqueduct of Sylvius, preventing cerebrospinal fluid (CSF) outflow from the ventricles and leading to hydrocephalus. This produces signs of increased intracranial pressure, namely papilledema, headache, nausea, and vomiting.

The ocular symptoms are part of an entity known as <u>Parinaud's syndrome</u>, which occurs with compression of the superior colliculus and pretectal area of the mesencephalon. Parinaud's syndrome consists of varying degrees of <u>impairment of conjugate upgaze and ocular convergence</u> along with pupillary abnormalities. Other associated symptoms include retractory nystagmus, convergence spasms, and upper lid retraction. Further compression of the brain stem caudally can lead to impaired downgaze as well.

2.   Although they account for only 0.4 to 1% of all intracranial tumors, pineal region tumors represent a broad histological spectrum. These tumors can be classified into four groups:

    1.   <u>Tumors of germ cell origin</u>
        a) benign: teratoma, dermoid
        b) malignant: germinoma, embryonal cell carcinoma, teratocarcinoma

    2.   <u>Tumors of pineal parenchymal cells:</u> pineocytoma, pineoblastoma

    3.   <u>Tumors of glial cells</u>: astrocytoma, glioblastoma, ependymoma, oligodendroglioma

    4.   <u>Miscellaneous</u>: meningioma, metastases, chorid plexus papilloma, hemangioblastoma, chemodectoma, sarcoma, benign cysts

Glial cell tumors and germinomas are the most common tumors in this region. Germinomas tend to occur in adolescence and have a strong predilection for men. Up to one third of glial cell tumors are low grade astrocytomas which have a high rate of surgical cure.

3. Computed tomography (CT) scans are invaluable for estimating the size and position of tumor, the degree of hydrocephalus, and the presence of calcific, cystic, or hemorrhagic components. MRI with sagittal and coronal views is helpful for further defining the tumor's anatomical boundaries. Angiography is not necessary unless a vascular abnormality is suspected.

A preoperative lumbar puncture to obtain CSF for cytology and tumor markers is indicated if there is no intracranial hypertension. CSF cytology may give an indication of tumor histology. Alpha fetoprotein and beta human chorionic gonadotropin are tumor markers that, if present, can be measured in serum or CSF. Elevated alpha fetoprotein levels are associated with endodermal sinus tumors, embryonal carcinomas, and some immature teratomas. Beta human chorionic gonadotropin can be elevated in embryonal cell carcinomas, germinomas, and malignant teratomas.

4. Although some controversy exists, the current consensus is that surgery is indicated for all tumors of the pineal region. Most neurosurgeons prefer an infratentorial, supracerebellar approach. Benign tumors should be pursued aggressively to achieve a gross total removal and optimize chances for a surgical cure. Even if a tumor is malignant, and total resection is not feasible due to invasiveness of vital structures, surgery is necessary for debulking the tumor and obtaining an accurate histological identification. Tumor histology is crucial for properly directing postoperative chemotherapy and radiation treatment.

Because many pineal region tumors are radiosensitive, many surgeons advocate a stereotactic needle biopsy with subsequent radiotherapy. There are several drawbacks to this approach including high risk of uncontrollable bleeding, inability to debulk tumors, and difficulty in making histological identification in a small tissue sample. Furthermore, if the tumor is benign, the patient will require an open procedure to remove the remaining tumor. Improved surgical techniques have resulted in lower mortality and morbidity rates, justifying aggressive surgery in these patients.

5. Most malignant tumors are radiosensitive to at least some degree and radiotherapy is indicated. The most radiosensitive tumors are germinomas and pineal parenchymal tumors. Chemotherapy is more controversial but may prove to be effective in recurrent germinomas, choriocarcinomas, embryonal cell carcinomas, and teratocarcinomas.

6. Patients with hydrocephalus prior to tumor removal will require measures to control increased intracranial pressure. Usually a ventriculoperational shunt is placed several days before surgery to permit a gradual reduction of ventricular size and pressure. Alternatively a ventricular drain can be placed at the time of surgery. This drain can be removed or converted to a shunt several days after surgery depending on the patient's postoperative requirements.

PEARLS:

1. Up to 30% of pineal region tumors are benign and amenable to surgical cure.

2. A small but significant number of patients present with endocrine disorders through involvement of the hypothalamus and anterior third ventricle. The most common endocrine manifestations of the pineal tumors are diabetes insipidus, precocious puberty, and various pituitary disorders.

PITFALLS:

1. Tumor seeding through the CSF pathways usually involves the spinal cord. This occurs most commonly with germinomas but any malignant pineal tumor is capable of seeding. CT myelography is

indicated for patients having a tumor with seeding potential. Spinal radiotherapy is indicated when seeding is present.

2. Occasionally, tumors are of a mixed cell type, containing elements of two or more cell lines. Therefore careful attention must be paid to examination of all tissue specimens. This is further rationale for avoiding stereotactic biopsies where tissue sampling is limited.

3. Vascular abnormalities are rare but can occur in this region. A high suspicion must be maintained, particularly when increased contrast enhancement is present on CT scan. Angiography will identify arteriovenous malformations, vein of Galen malformations, and aneurysms.

REFERENCES

1. Chapman PH, Linggood RM: The management of pineal area tumors: a recent reappraisal. Cancer 46:1253-1257, 1980.

2. Neuwelt EA, ed.:   Diagnosis and Treatment of Pineal Region Tumors. Williams & Wilkins, Baltimore, 1984.

3. Reid WS, Clark WK: Comparison of the infratentorial and transtentorial approaches to the pineal region. Neurosurgery 3:1-8,1978.

4. Rubinstein LJ: Cytogenesis and differentiation of pineal neoplasms. Human Pathol 12:441-447, 1981.

5. Stein BM: Supracerebellar approach for pineal region neoplasms in Schmidek HH, Sweet WH, ed. Operative neurosurgical techniques. Grune and Stratton, New York, 1982, pp 599-607.

6. Stein BM, Fetell MR: Therapeutic modalities for pineal region tumors.   Clinical Neurosurg 32:445-455, 1985.

RAPIDLY PROGRESSIVE SPINAL CORD DYSFUNCTION

CASE 22: A 44-year-old man who underwent a right nephrectomy for renal cell carcinoma 1 year prior to admission presented with lower thoracic back pain. Metastatic workup at the time of his nephrectomy was unremarkable. Nine months prior to his current presentation he began to have localized, nonradiating pain in this lower thoracic region. His pain initially responded to analgesics but gradually became more severe. Three days prior to admission he began to have difficulty walking due to a sense of heaviness in both legs. He had constipation for approximately 2 weeks with some recent urinary hesitancy. When he awoke on the day of admission he was unable to walk.

On examination his mental status and cranial nerves were intact. There was some localized tenderness to fist percussion over the lower thoracic vertebrae. There was weakness in both legs although they could be lifted against moderate resistance. He was able to stand unaided but could not walk without assistance. Sensory examination revealed decreased pinprick and light touch sensation extending down from the pubis. Vibratory and position sense were intact. Decreased rectal tone was present on rectal examination. Deep1 tendon reflexes were increased in the lower extremities with a present Babinski sign bilaterally. A urinary catheter was introduced and revealed a postvoid residual of 250 ml of urine (consistent with neurogenic bladder).

Neuroanatomical Clue:

An emergency spinal x-ray series and myelogram were obtained. The myelogram on the opposite page demonstrates an epidural mass compressing the cord from the lower margin of T11 to the upper margin of L1.

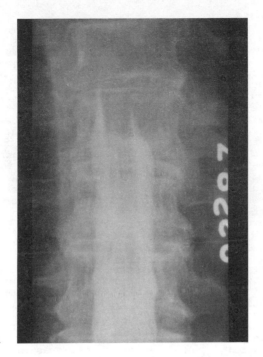

Figure 22.1

QUESTIONS:

1. What is the diagnosis?

2. What are the most common histological types of this tumor?

3. What radiological studies are helpful in the workup?

4. What is the role of radiotherapy in treating this tumor?

5. What are the indications for surgery?

6. What are the main factors influencing the recovery of function?

ANSWERS:

1. By far the most common diagnosis of a spinal epidural mass is a metastatic tumor. In fact metastatic tumor is the most common type of neoplasm in the spinal canal. Some benign tumors such as neurilemmomas, neurofibromas and meningiomas may have extradural components although they are generally intradural. Given this patient's history of renal cell carcinoma, metastasis to the thoracic vertebrae is likely. The symptoms of bilateral motor weakness, bladder and bowel dysfunction, localized pain, increased deep tendon reflex, and sensory deficits are all indicative of spinal cord dysfunction. The loss of light touch and pinprick sensation with preservation of vibratory and position sense imply anterior (ventral) cord compression with lesser involvement of the dorsal columns.

2. Lung cancer, breast cancer, and lymphoma are responsible for approximately one half of all spinal metastases. The remainder are mostly split between genitourinary and gastrointestinal malignancies and multiple myeloma. In 5 to 10% of patients the primary malignancy cannot be found.

    Autopsy series show that although breast cancer, lung cancer, and lymphoma accounted for the majority of spinal metastasis, they had considerably less of a propensity to seed than other types of tumors. Tumors with the highest propensity included multiple myeloma, prostatic carcinoma, and renal carcinoma.

3. Initial workup should consist of complete plain x-rays of the entire spine to screen for multifocal involvement which is present 20% of the time. Plain film abnormalities include osteolytic or osteoblastic bony changes, pathological compression fractures, pedicle destruction, or scalloping of vertebral bodies.

Myelography is the most important test for determining the extent of tumor involvement and the presence of multifocal lesions. Epidural lesions tend to produce an hourglass deformity if partial block is present, and a tapering paint brush appearance with a complete block. A computed tomography (CT) scan is helpful following myelography to provide detail in areas of abnormality.

Studies with magnetic resonance imaging (MRI) are preliminary, but suggest that with experience it will become an important diagnostic modality. Spinal angiography has not proven to be of benefit.

4. Radiotherapy and surgical decompression are the main treatment modalities, however, a great deal of controversy surrounds their use. Current evidence seems to indicate that radiotherapy is the primary mode of treatment in patients presenting with spinal metastases. With some important exceptions radiotherapy appears to be more effective than surgery alone, and equally as effective as a combined radiotherapy and surgical approach. The most radiosensitive tumors are lymphomas and myelomas. In tumors that are radioresistant a trial of radiotherapy is usually indicated provided the neurological deficit is not severe and rapidly progressive.

5. Although radiotherapy is considered the initial treatment modality, there are several indications for surgery:

    1. Failure to respond to radiotherapy - usually with progressive decline in neurological function

    2. Spinal instability or compression by bone-Spinal instability or pathological fractures often require decompression and spinal fusion.

3. Radioresistant tumor - When the tumor is known to be radioresistant, surgery is often the primary mode of therapy particularly when significant neurological dysfunction is present.

4. Previous spinal cord irradiation - with tumor occurrence in areas where further radiotherapy would exceed spinal cord tolerance for irradiation

5. Unknown diagnosis - when etiology of mass is unknown and tissue diagnosis is needed

6. Repeat surgical decompression for recurrent tumor - reoperation for relapse occurring after previous surgical decompression

6. Prognosis is closely associated with pretreatment neurological status. Patients who are able to walk before treatment have a much better prognosis than patients who are paraplegic or have bladder and bowel involvement. A worse prognosis is also associated with rapid onset and rapid progression of neurological deficits. More favorable prognosis is associated with myeloma, lymphoma, breast cancer and prostate cancer compared to bronchogenic carcinoma, melanoma, and soft tissue sarcoma. Vertebral collapse carries a less favorable prognosis.

PEARLS:

1. Although spinal metastasis usually occurs in patients with a known primary tumor, in 5-10% of patients spinal cord compression from a metastatic tumor represents the initial manifestation of a malignancy.

2. Pain is often the initial symptom (more than 90% of cases) in patients with spinal metastases. It often precedes other symptoms by days to years.

3. Steroids and/or mannitol are useful adjuncts to
    treating these tumors on a short term basis.   The
    beneficial effect is probably mediated through a
    reduction in cord edema.

4. Extraspinal malignancies are believed to spread to
    the extradural space mainly by hematogenous spread
    through   Batson's   plexus,   an   extradural,
    paravertebral venous plexus.

PITFALLS:

1. A high index of suspicion must be maintained in
    patients known to have cancer.   It is important to
    make the diagnosis as early as possible to be able
    to preserve neurological function.   Patients have a
    median duration of symptoms of 2 months before
    diagnosis is made.

2. A tumor located in the anterior portion of the
    epidural space is less favorable than one located
    laterally or posteriorly.   Anterior tumors require
    an anterior approach to the spine which is more
    complicated and associated with higher morbidity.
    Posterior and lateral tumors can usually be
    decompressed through a simple laminectomy.

3. It is crucial that rehabilitation begin as soon as
    the clinical condition allows in patients with
    neurological deficits.   This involves physical
    therapy, bowel, bladder, and skin care, and
    training to permit independence in daily care
    activities.

4. When a complete block is demonstrated on a
    myelogram where the dye has been introduced below
    the level of the block, the upper extent of the
    lesion is generally not known.   This may require
    the instillation of dye above the level of the
    block by a C1 puncture to completely define the
    number of levels over which the lesion extends.

REFERENCES

1. Black P: Spinal metastasis: current status and recommended guidelines for management. Neurosurgery 5:726-746, 1979.

2. Black P: Spinal epidural tumors, In Wilkins RH, Rengachary SS, eds: Neurosurgery McGraw-Hill Co., New York, 1985, pp 1062-1069.

3. Gilbert RW, Kim JH, Posner JB: Epidural spinal cord compression from metastatic tumor: diagnosis and treatment. Ann Neurol 3:40-51, 1978.

4. Livingston K, Perrin R: The neurosurgical management of spinal metastases causing cord and cauda equina compression. J Neurosurg 49:839-843, 1978.

5. Tomaszek DE, Mahaley MS: Management of spinal epidural metastases. Contemp Neurosurg 5:1-6, 1983.

6. Ushio Y, Posner R, Posner J, et al: Experimental spinal cord compression by epidural neoplasm. Neurology (Minneapolis) 27:422-429, 1971.

FAILURE TO THRIVE AND INCREASING HEAD SIZE IN AN INFANT

CASE 23: A 1-year-old male child presented with a 6 month history of irritability, lethargy, and increasing head size. Examination revealed an enlarged head with splayed sutures and a bulging open fontanelle. The child also had poor upgaze and bilateral VIth nerve palsies. A computed tomography (CT) scan was obtained.

Clue:

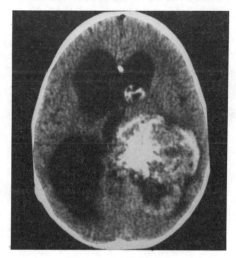

Figure 23.1   CT scan of head

QUESTIONS:

1. Describe the findings and location of this lesion on the CT scan. How do these findings explain the child's presentation?

2. What is the likely diagnosis in this case? What other tumors are found within the ventricles?

3. What is the etiology of the hydrocephalus?

4. What is the treatment of this condition and what complications could be encountered?

131

ANSWERS:

1.   There are 2 important findings on this CT scan.
     The first is the presence of a large inhomogenously
     contrast-enhancing mass on the right side.   The
     mass is surrounding by the cerebrospinal fluid
     (CSF) of the lateral ventricle and therefore this
     tumor is intraventricular in location.   The portion
     of the ventricle involved is the atrium of the
     lateral ventricle, or that curved portion of the
     lateral ventricular system between the body and
     temporal horn of the lateral ventricle.   The second
     important finding is a marked dilation of the
     entire ventricular system that represents
     hydrocephalus in this child.

     The hydrocephalus demonstrated on the scan is
     responsible for this clinical presentation.
     Hydrocephalus in children before the age of 1 year
     will cause splitting and nonfusion of the cranial
     sutures as well as bulging of the anterior
     fontanelle secondary to chronic and progressively
     increasing intracranial pressure.   The bilateral
     VIth nerve palsies and poor upgaze are also signs
     of hydrocephalus in children and are felt to be
     secondary either to traction on the nerves from
     increased pressure or dorsal midbrain pressure from
     a dilated IIIrd ventricle.   The nausea, vomiting,
     and headache frequently associated with increased
     intracranial pressure in children results in a
     failure to thrive with irritability and poor
     feeding habits.

2.   The presence of a lateral intraventricular tumor
     with hydrocephalus in a young child strongly
     suggests the diagnosis of a choroid plexus
     papilloma.   This is usually a benign, slow growing
     tumor that originates from the epithelial cells
     that cover the ventricular choroid plexus.   The
     tumor occurs in all age groups but 70% are found in
     patients less than 2 years of age and they are most
     commonly located in the lateral ventricle.   The
     most common primary intraventricular tumor in
     children is the ependymoma which is most frequently
     located in the IVth ventricle.   Primary brain
     astroglial neoplasms which may project into any of

the ventricles are subependymomas, astrocytomas, glioblastomas, medulloblastomas, and pineal region tumors (IIIrd ventricle).

In adults, benign cysts are encountered and include the colloid cyst of the anterior IIIrd ventricle, dermoids, epidermoids, and craniopharyngiomas. Meningiomas are also found intraventricularly, primarly in the older age groups, and are thought to arise from arachnoidal cells in the choroid plexus.

3. The etiology of hydrocephalus in children with choroid plexus papillomas is not known but many theories have been proposed. One is that choroid plexus papillomas are known to produce CSF and therefore the hydrocephalus is secondary to the over-production of CSF (primary hydrocephalus).

   Another mechanism is the obstruction of CSF pathways by the tumor itself. This is likely to occur only with very large tumors that are located either in the IIIrd or IVth ventricles (obstructive hydrocephalus). Absorption of CSF may also be blocked from repeated small hemorrhages from the tumor as the breakdown products of these bleeds impairs the flow and diffusion of CSF across the arachnoid villi (communicating hydrocephalus).

4. The treatment of choice for choroid plexus papillomas is complete surgical resection. When this tumor is located in the atrium of the lateral ventricle, no approach is completely satisfactory when trying to balance protection of the surrounding brain with complete removal of the tumor. Approaches through the superior parietal lobule or temporal and occipital lobes may be used. Because these tumors are quite vascular, receiving blood supply from both the anterior and posterior choroidal arteries, the control of blood loss is of particular importance in young children.

   Postoperative complications include seizures, intraventricular hemorrhage, hydrocephalus, and bilateral subdural hematomas. Not all patients will require shunting after complete resection of a choroid plexus papilloma although the majority will because of preexisting communicating hydrocephalus. Subdural hematomas and hygromas occur when the greatly dilated ventricles are rapidly collapsed during shunting or surgery and may require drainage or direct shunting if symptomatic postoperatively.

PEARLS:

1.   Choroid plexus papillomas are more frequent in the IVth ventricle than the lateral ventricle in adults.   The reverse situation is true for children.

2.   Intraventricular tumors are more common in children that adults and usually involve the IVth ventricle.

3.   Always consider the spread of tumor cells through the CSF pathways in patients with intraventricular tumors.   Some patients will require a myelogram or magnetic resonance imaging (MRI) to rule out spinal spread or "drop metastasis" from their tumors, especially ependymomas of the IVth ventricle.

PITFALLS:

1.   Occasionally choroid plexus tumors may be malignant.   These tumors may seed the CSF pathways and have median survival times of only 2-3 years.

2.   Twenty percent of childhood choroid plexus papillomas demonstrated signs of malignant degeneration, especially before the age of 2 years.

3.   Tumors involving or projecting into the ventricles may seed tumor cells through shunt systems.   This may lead to the hematogenous or pertoneal spread of tumor cells, particularly medulloblastomas and pineal region neoplasms.

REFERENCES

1. Boyd M, Steinbok P: Choroid plexus tumors:
   problems in diagnosis and management.   J Neurosurg
   66:800-805, 1987.

2. Carpenter DB, Michelsen WJ, Mays AP: Carcinara of
   the choroid plexus. Case Report. J Neurosurg 56:
   722-727, 1982.

3. Laurence KM: The biology of choroid plexus papillae
   in infancy and childhood.   Acta Neuro Chir 50:79-
   90, 1979.

4. Matsar DD, Croftin FD: Papillae of the choroid
   plexus in childhood. J Neurosurg 17:1002-1026, 1960.

5. Thompson JR: Harwood-Nash DC, Fitz CR: The
   neuroradiology   of   childhood   choroid   plexus
   neoplasms. AJR 118:116-133, 1973.

PROGRESSIVE LETHARGY, SLURRED SPEECH, AND HEMIPARESIS IN AN ELDERLY ALCOHOLIC

CASE 24: This 75-year-old man with a history of alcohol abuse and known hepatic cirrhosis was evaluated for lethargy and slurred speech. The patient's family had noted progressive drowsiness for 1 week. The evening prior to admission the patient fell and may have struck his head on the floor. Following his fall he became more sleepy and his speech became slurred.

On examination the patient was lethargic and unable to follow simple commands. He verbalized but in an unintelligible fashion. His pupils were equal and reactive bilaterally. The remainder of his cranial nerve examination was unremarkable. He demonstrated a mild right hemiparesis and hyperreflexia. His initial laboratory values included a prothrombin time of 14.6 seconds with 12.0 seconds as control. His total bilirubin was mildly elevated as was his ammonia level.

Neuroanatomical Clue: Computed tomography (CT) scan of the head

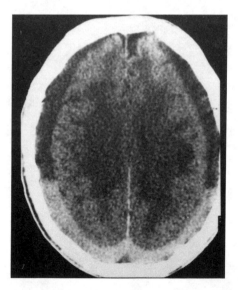

Figure 24.1

QUESTIONS:

1. What historical points and findings on examination
   are characteristic of patients with chronic subdural
   hematomas?

2. What are the characteristic findings on CT scan?

3. Which patients are treated and what are the
   approaches to therapy?

4. List several complications associated with chronic
   subdural hematomas and their treatment?

ANSWERS:

1. Although the overall incidence of <u>chronic subdural hematomas</u> has been estimated at 1-2/100,000 population, the incidence increases severalfold in those patients over 50 years of age. Mean ages of occurrence have been reported from 56 to 63. The fact that the patient described above has a history of chronic alcoholism is an important predisposing factor. <u>Coagulopathies or anticoagulation and epilepsy are other significant risk factors</u>. The lack of a history of significant head trauma is not uncommon. In 25-50% of patients with chronic subdural hematomas, no such history can be obtained. Even when a history of trauma exists, it is often, as here, very mild in nature.

    <u>Impaired consciousness and hemiparesis</u> are the two most frequent signs of chronic subdural hematomas occurring in approximately 53 and 45% of patients, respectively. Other important although nonspecific signs include other mental status changes, papilledema, dysphasia, IIIrd nerve palsies, and hemianopsias. Because of such findings and the lack of significant trauma history, chronic subdural hematomas commonly are misdiagnosed initially as dementia, strokes, or brain tumors.

2. The appearance of a subdural hematoma on a CT scan changes with the age of the hematoma. <u>Those under 1 week old are hyperdense. Between 7 and 21 days subdurals are generally isodense in comparison with brain. Subdurals greater than 3 weeks of age are usually hypodense</u> although with chronic rebleeding they often demonstrate different zones of densities. In this patient the chronic, hypodense fluid is seen anteriorly while the more acute component of the hematoma has layered posteriorly. Chronic subdurals classically are crescent shaped with effacement of the underlying sulci and often ventricular compression as well. In unilateral hematomas, midline structures are frequently shifted. In bilateral hematomas, however, midline shift may not be present. Displacement of the gray-white junction medially should secure the

diagnosis. Also contrast may be administered which may enhance the membranes surrounding the hematoma. The outer membrane forms during the first week and the inner membrane forms after approximately 3 weeks.

3. All symptomatic patients should be treated. Successful medical therapy has been reported. Unfortunately this usually entails several weeks of bed rest for immobilization, accompanied by prolonged courses of diuretics and steroids with their attendant risks. Furthermore, during this period the patient remains at risk for sudden neurological deterioration. Therefore, surgery is the treatment of choice. Craniotomy has been used in the past to afford wider exposure and allow removal of membranes and any solid components. The recognition of several factors limits the need for craniotomy. First these hematomas are mostly liquid and often can be drained through smaller openings. Second there is no improvement in outcome associated with removal of the membranes. Last, sudden decompression and drainage with craniotomy has occasionally been associated with neurological deterioration. Because of this, drainage via burr holes or twist drill craniostomy is now standard therapy in most cases. Most liquid subdurals may be drained by a single burr hole placed over the area of maximal thickness of the clot. Occasionally a second burr hole is used for irrigation in those hematomas with solid components. Generally, a drain is left in the subdural space for 24 hours post operatively to provide evacuation of residual hematoma. Twist drill aspiration is another alternative surgical therapy which may be performed under local anesthesia with minimal surgical trauma. In this procedure a hole is placed with a twist drill at a 45° angle to the skull. A small catheter is then placed in the subdural space and attached to close, gravity drainage. The hematoma is gradually siphoned off over the next 24 hours.

4. Residual hematoma is extremely common in treated chronic subdural hematoma. In general, complete removal is not required to produce clinical improvement and eventual resorption.

    Actual reaccumulation occurs in 8-45% of cases and should be suspected if a patient deteriorates or fails to improve postoperatively. Reaccumulation is more common following craniotomy than burr hole or twist drill drainage. In cases of bilateral hematomas, both must be removed to prevent rapid shift of midline structures and resulting neurological deterioration. Sudden deterioration has also been sporadically associated with too rapid evacuation of clot. Seizures occur in approximately 10% of patients and prophylactic anticonvulsants are indicated. Finally, infections occur in less than 1% of patients with chronic subdural hematoma and include subdural empyema, brain abscess, meningitis, and bone flap infection.

PEARLS:

1. Outcome is most closely correlated to the patients preoperative neurological status. Overall mortality is less than 10%. Thirteen percent of patients who are initially comatose or stuporous expire whereas only 5% of those initially alert or drowsy die. As many as 75% of patients may be expected to return to their normal functional level.

2. Bilateral subdurals are generally reported to be present in 15 to 20% of patients. Their associated mortality is similar to unilateral chronic subdurals.

3. Angiographically, chronic subdural hematomas appear as avascular masses between the inner table of the skull and the surface of the cortex on the anteroposterior (AP) view. With diagnostic accuracy of 99% this was the most important modality for evaluation prior to CT scanning.

PITFALLS:

1. Lack of consideration of the diagnosis is a major problem. With their often insidious onset and non-specific symptoms and signs chronic subdural hematomas have been misdiagnosed in as many as 40% of patients' admitting diagnoses, prior to the wide availability of CT scanning.

REFERENCES

1. Carmel M, Grubb RL: Treatment of chronic subdural hematoma by twist-drill craniostomy with continuous catheter drainage. J Neurosurg 65:183-187, 1986.

2. Cooper PR: Posttraumatic intracranial mass lesions. In Cooper PR, ed. Head injury. Baltimore, Williams & Wilkins, 1982, pp 185-232.

3. Markwalder TM: Chronic subdural hematomas: a review. J Neurosurg 54:637-645, 1981.

4. McKissock W, Richardson A, Bloom WH: Subdural hematoma: a review of 389 cases. Lancet 1:1365-1369, 1960.

5. Tabaddor K, Shulman K: Definitive treatment of chronic subdural hematoma by twist-drill craniostomy and closed system drainage. J Neurosurg 46:220-226, 1977.

JUMPING VISION, UNSTEADINESS OF GAIT

CASE 25: A 22-year-old woman presented with the complaint of "jumping vision." In addition, she noted trouble with walking, headaches, weakness, and "muscle cramps" of her legs. On examination, she had prominent downbeat nystagmus, which was aggravated by downward gaze. Her gait was broad-based, and she was noted to have weakness throughout. Her reflexes were hyperactive, with upgoing toes bilaterally. Her speech was palatal. With the constellation of symptoms representing the foramen magnum compression syndrome, she underwent a myelogram including the posterior fossa which showed a filling defect in the upper cervical region. This was consistent with a downward displacement of the cerebellar tonsils through the foramen magnum and a posteriorly displaced and kinked brain stem.

Neuroanatomical Clue:

   Compression in the region of the medulla and foramen magnum disrupts multiple modalities both in neuroanatomical structures which originate here as well as pathways which cross this region. The involvement of the upper motor neurons (spastic paresis) and proprioceptive fibers (ataxia) place the lesion below the pons, while the palatal speech and oscillopsia implicate the lower cranial nerve nuclei and the cerebellum.

Magnetic resonance imaging (MRI) of Chiari malformation
(CM) junction:

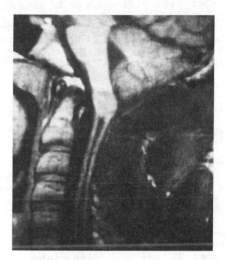

Figure 25.1

QUESTIONS:

1. What is the most likely diagnosis in this case?
   What are other types of lesions that could present
   with similar findings?

2. The abnormality in this case presented with s i g n s
   and   symptoms   consistent   with   foramen   magnum
   compression.   What are the other symptoms that may
   be associated with this lesion?

3. What   findings   on   various   neuroradiological
   procedures would help to confirm the diagnosis?

4. What is the surgical approach to this lesion?

5. The   Arnold-Chiari   malformation   represents   the
   mildest form of a spectrum of disorders involving
   the brain stem, cerebellum, and craniocervical
   junction.   What are the important features of the
   various types of Chiari malformations?

ANSWERS:

1. The most likely diagnosis is an <u>Arnold Chiari "Type I" Malformation</u>. The patient in this Case Study presented with findings consistent with foramen magnum compression. Other processes that may mimic this presentation are tumors of the skull base and foramen magnum, such as meningiomas and chordomas.

    As will be seen in the next question, the Arnold-Chiari malformation bears a variety of presenting symptoms. Other lesions which must be considered include intramedullary processes, such as syringomyelia, tumor and hemangioma, as well as demyelinating diseases such as multiple sclerosis.

2. In a large clinical series, 30% of the patients with Arnold-Chiari malformations presented with a <u>foramen magnum compression syndrome</u>, as did the woman in this Case Study. Twenty-two percent of patients presented with paroxysmal, intracranial hypertension (exertional headache, nausea/vomiting, dizziness, blurred vision), 20% with a central cord syndrome (pain, dissociated sensory loss, weakness), 10% with cerebellar dysfunction (gait, truncal or limb ataxia, nystagmus, dysarthria), and the remainder with either spasticity or bulbar palsy.

3. Although not diagnostic for Arnold Chiari, 40-50% of plain cervical and skull films will reveal an associated anomaly, such as <u>basilar impression, atlantooccipital fusion, or spina bifida occulta</u>. Myelogram reveals a posterior filling defect, sometimes seen to be bilobed, extending into the cervical region. Arteriography, while rarely used nowadays, may reveal displacement of the posterior inferior cerebellar arteries through the foramen magnum. Computed tomographic (CT) scan following metrizamide myelogram reveals inferior displacement of the cerebellar tonsils into the upper cervical region. The definite studies are provided by <u>magnetic resonance imaging</u> (MRI), which allows better anatomical definition of the posterior fossa and upper cervical regions. This clearly shows the

inferior herniation of the cerebellar tonsils, as well as any associated abnormalities of the midbrain and cerebellum.

4. The goal of surgery is decompression of the foramen magnum and upper cervical cord. The patient may be either seated or prone during surgery. The posterior rim of the foramen magnum is removed, and a limited cervical laminectomy is performed. If necessary, the outflow of the fourth ventricle is restored. A dural patch is sewn into place to increase the cross-sectional area of the dural sac in this region and any thickening of the dura around the foramen magnum is incised to allow sufficient relaxation of the dura to release pressure on neural structures.

5. The Arnold-Chiari malformation, also known as the Chiari Type I or "adult" form, consists of variable caudal displacement of the cerebellar tonsils without displacement of the medulla. This form typically presents in the fifth decade of life.

    The Chiari II or "child" form consists of variable caudal displacement of the vermis, pons, and medulla, as well as elongation of the fourth ventricle. This form presents early in life, may require shunting for relief of hydrocephalus, and is associated with respiratory embarrassment.

    The Chiari III malformation consists of caudal displacement of the medulla and herniation of the cerebellum into the cervical canal, and myleomeningocoele.

    The Chiari IV malformation consists of cerebellar hypoplasia but is considered by most to be unrelated to the other types mentioned above.

PEARLS:

1. There is a strong association of syringomyelia with the Arnold-Chiari malformation - as many as 75% of patients presenting with a Chiari I malformation will have an associated syrinx. These data were obtained from series collected before MRI became

available.   As MRI is extremely sensitive for syringomyelia, it is possible that an even greater percentage of Chiari patients will be found to have associated syrinx.

2. Regardless of presenting complaints, 75% of patients will be found to have lower extremity hyperreflexia - the most common sign. Forty to 60% of patients will show some sensory loss, slowed alternating movements, nystagmus, and gait ataxia on careful neurological examination.

3. Ten percent of patients will have a normal neurological examination, and will have an occipital headache as their only symptom.

4. There is an <u>association of both birth trauma and meningitis with Arnold Chiari malformation</u>. Some authors have postulated that these processes lead to local adhesions and cerebrospinal fluid (CSF) blockage which in turn leads to tonsillar herniation.

5. <u>Thirty-three percent of patients with downbeat nystagmus will have an abnormality at the craniocervical junction</u>, particularly Arnold-Chiari malformation.

PITFALLS:

1. Extensive cervical laminectomies, particularly in children, put the patient at risk for spinal deformities. Decompression should be limited to those levels where absolutely necessary, and patients must be carefully followed postoperatively.

2. <u>Adhesions</u> may be an etiological factor in the development of the Arnold-Chiari malformation, so care must be taken intraoperatively, not to risk increased adhesion formation.

3. For optimal outcome, the circulation of the fourth ventricle and the craniospinal junction must be restored to a normal pattern.

REFERENCES

1. Appleby A, Foster JB, Hankinson J, et al: The diagnosis and management of the Chiari anomalic in adult life. Brain 91:131-140, 1968.

2. Carmel PW, Markesbery WR: Early descriptions of the Arnold-Chiari malformation. J Neurosurg 37:543-547, 1972.

3. Oakes WJ: Chiari malformation hydromyelia, syringomyelia. In Wilkins and Rengarchary, eds. Neurosurgery, New York, McGraw Hill Book Co., 1985.

4. Paul KS, Iye RH, Stray FA, et al: Arnold-Chiari malformation. J Neurosurg 58:183-187, 1983.

5. Saey RT, Onofrio BM, Youagihara T: Experience with Arnold-Chiari malformation; 1960-1970. J Neurosurg 45:416-422, 1976.

6. Wellch K, Shillito J, Strand R, et al: Chiari I "Malformation" - an acquired disorder? J Neurosurg 55:604-609, 1981.

FAILED BACK SYNDROME - ARACHNOIDITIS, STIMULATORS, MORPHINE PUMP

CASE 26: A 38-year-old man presented with low back and leg pain. After a fall 10 years ago, he complained of severe low back pain that radiated down his right leg (L5 distribution). Symptoms resolved with bed rest, but 2 years later he underwent L45 laminectomy and discectomy with excellent pain relief. Similar symptoms recurred 1 year later and the patient underwent a decompressive lumbar laminectomy and fusion for spinal stenosis. The patient again did well postoperatively for about 1 year and then noted recurrent low back pain with radiation into both legs (R>L) and occasional paresthesias. He again participated in an extensive conservative treatment rehabilitation program, including medications (e.g., tricyclic antidepressants, major tranquilizers, and antiinflammatory analgesics), physical therapy, psychotherapy, acupuncture, and transcutaneous electrical nerve stimulation (TENS) therapy. The patient's pain continued and he became addicted to narcotics. Throughout most of these years, the patient was able to continue his work but with a progressive decline in work time. The patient then presented for neurosurgical evaluation, complaining of "horrible, constant pain" in his lower back and both legs (R>L) that increased with sitting, standing, or walking.

Examination revealed lumbosacral paraspinous spasm with severe limitation of bending and a stiff deliberate gait. Straight leg raising was positive on the right at 25° and the left at 70°. A mild hypesthesia was present below L5 bilaterally (R>L). No definite weakness was detected, but ankle reflexes were diminished (R>L). Plain x-rays detected no abnormal motion and electromyograph (EMG) revealed no active changes. A myelogram was consistent with arachnoiditis and epidural fibrosis, without evidence of compression.

QUESTIONS:

1. What is the "failed back syndrome"?

2. What is the failure rate of operations for lumbar
   root decompression?

3. What neuroaugmentative devices are useful in
   the treatment of this syndrome?

4. Is there a role for narcotic analgesics
   (systemic   or   intraspinal)   in   the   treatment   of
   benign chronic pain?

ANSWERS:

1. <u>The failed back syndrome (FBS) can be defined as
    "the failure of surgical or medical therapy to
    relieve pain and incapacitation from low back or
    leg pain."</u> Disabling low back pain (LBP) is the
    single most common medical complaint in the United
    States.   Approximately 3 of every 4 people
    experience a disabling episode of lumbago   or
    sciatica in their lifetime.   Chronic LBP is a
    complaint of about 20% of adults and is responsible
    for   chronic disability in about 10%.   At any one
    time this would represent about 18,000,000 people
    and accounts for 1/6 of all hospital bed days. <u>In
    1984, LBP was estimated to have cost $21 billion
    for medical care</u>, compensation, and litigation
    (excluding loss of productivity).   In some
    patients, the FBS is felt to   have an organic
    basis.   This would include lateral and central
    spinal   stenosis and persistent or recurrent
    herniated nucleus pulposus [decreasing with high
    resolution computed tomography (CT) scanning],
    adhesive arachnoiditis   (decreasing with CT
    replacing myelography in many cases and the use of
    better   tolerated   contrast   agents),   epidural
    fibrosis (decreased by using autogenous fat
    grafts), chronic mechanical pain, nerve injury
    (i.e., during surgery, causalgia), intraneural
    fibrosis, spondylolysis or spondylolisthesis above
    a fusion, pseudoarthrosis, foreign body, or rarely
    operation at the   wrong level or side.   Thus, a
    number of the patients diagnosed initially with
    this syndrome will be found to harbor a surgically
    remediable abnormality.   However, a large number
    of patients remain with a complex and often severe
    health problem and when considering surgery it must
    be kept in mind that some of these diagnoses are
    actually caused by surgery. Nonorganic factors are
    a critical aspect of FBS and include psychological,
    drug, social, and financial factors. Chronic pain
    commonly results in the "chronic pain syndrome,"
    involving hysteria, depression, anxiety, and
    hypochondriasis. A multidisciplinary approach
    combining the knowledge and experience of
    neurology, psychiatry, rehabilitation medicine,
    neurosurgery, and orthopedics is best able to
    manage these difficult patients.   The objective is

to accurately diagnose and treat (if possible) any organic problems and then to alleviate pain as much as possible (safely), while addressing the contributing factors and maximizing the patient's functional capacity. Psychotherapy, often including the pharmacological treatment of depression (tricyclic antidepressants) and/or anxiety (with major tranquilizers, not benzodiazepines), and an active rehabilitation program are key aspects of any treatment program. Weight loss, behavior modification and education for appropriate expectations are also important factors in the overall treatment of the "failed back."

2. Failure rates following operation for low back pain with radiculopathy vary between 10 and 40%, with the overall rate probably being greater than 35% when all patients are included. Failure implies the persistence of severe radiating pain, not back pain alone. At least some "failures" are in patients who undergo surgery with no physical findings suggestive of nerve root compression and some have possibly had an inadequate diagnostic evaluation. Appropriate surgery does alleviate the symptoms of many patients with low back and leg pain.

Before surgery, consideration must be given to preventative measures (e.g., avoid activities known to aggravate spine disease), a full trial of conservative therapy, and the correlation of physical findings to the history and to adequate diagnostic studies. It is important to keep in mind that radiographic abnormalities of the spine occur in many asymptomatic patients. The reported incidence of surgically remediable lesions in FBS varies from <10 to >80%. Many patients in the latter group benefited from reoperation (83% objectively and 73% subjectively improved). Surgery for radiculopathy must be directed toward the alleviation of nerve root compression while minimizing the introduction of instability. Lumbar fusion plays a role in the treatment of "mechanical low back syndrome," but unfortunately it is difficult to select the patients who will benefit from this surgery.

Fusion might best be restricted to patients with symptoms strongly related to weight bearing and who respond to cast immobilization.

3. "Neuroaugmentation" refers to pain relief induced by nervous system stimulation. This therapy was developed   after Melzack and Wall presented their "gate control" theory of pain transmission (5). They discovered that activity in large diameter afferents (e.g., nonpain fibers) can diminish the activity along pain transmission pathways. Based on this phenomenon, two different neuroaugmentative devices have been used extensively in patients with FBS   without   surgically   remediable   lesions. Transcutaneous electrical nerve stimulators (TENS) are the simplest and safest of these 2 devices. Electrodes placed on the skin (generally near the site of pain) are stimulated by a portable impulse generator.   TENS clearly diminishes acute pain (e.g. postoperative) and in a group of selected FBS patients (those without psychiatric problems), 33% found it beneficial (4).   Benefit can   include   dramatic   subjective   and   often functional improvement. Most patients who find it effective for more than 1 month will continue to benefit for more than 1 year, although a delayed loss   of   effectiveness   has   occurred   in   some patients.   The   original   effect   is   usually   not regained following a temporary withdrawal of TENS therapy in these patients. The usual TENS mediated pain relief is generally not naloxone reversible, however, low frequency stimulated analgesia has been reversed by naloxone. Thus TENS may modify pain perception by two different mechanisms. TENS must be discontinued in some patients secondary to skin   irritation   or   breakdown   and   some   find   the external   electrodes   and   device   cumbersome   or uncomfortable.   These factors, or inadequate pain relief, often lead to the application of the second neuroaugmentative device, the epidural spinal cord stimulator   (ESCS).   A   thoracolumbar   epidural electrode can be placed percutaneously using local anesthesia and a modified large spinal needle. This exteriorized electrode can be used for a trial stimulation period (up to several days) prior to implantation. Implantation under local anesthesia

involves   anchoring   of   the   electrode   and
subcutaneous   placement   of   an   inconspicuous
programmable   impulse   generator.   A   portable
programmer   allows   the   periodic   adjustment   of
several   parameters   to   maximize   stimulation
effectiveness.   Potential   complications   include
mechanical   failure,   electrode   migration   (requiring
manipulation   or   reinsertion),   and   a   small   rate   of
infection   (requiring   temporary   or   permanent   removal
and   antibiotic   treatment).   No   serious
complications   have   been   reported.   The   best
candidates   for   ESCS   are   patients   with   FBS   who   had
maximal   "causal"   treatment   as   well   as   appropriate
drug,   behavior   modification,   physical   therapy,   and
at   least   some   response   to   TENS   treatment.   One
could   expect   about   75%   of   patients   to   undergo
implantation   after   a   period   of   trial   stimulation
and   about   50%   of   those   implanted   will   report
prolonged   subjective   pain   relief,   while   about   16%
will   return   to   work   and   normal   activity.   It   must
be   remembered   by   patient   and   doctor   that   the
objective   with   ESCS   is   pain   management   and   not
"cure."

A   third   method   of   neuroaugmentation   involves   the
production   of   <u>prolonged   analgesia   by   the   transient
stimulation   of   certain   deep   brain   areas</u>   (the
periventricular/periaqueductal   gray   matter).   This
analgesia   is   partially   mediated   by   the   activation
of   an   endogenous   opioid   neuronal   system   because   in
some   patients   it   can   be   blocked   by   naloxone.   It
probably   involves   the   activation   of   a   descending
system   that   inhibits   pain   transmission   in   the
spinal   cord   or   at   reticular   formation   relays.   The
brain   stimulating   electrode   can   be   introduced   under
local   anesthesia   via   a   small   twist   drill
craniotomy,   using   CT   stereotactic   guidance,   and   is
connected   to   an   implanted   impulse   generator.   The
most   common   complication   with   this   procedure   is
mechanical   failure,   however,   there   is   the   small
risk   of   a   serious   complication,   including   central
nervous   system   (CNS)   infection,   intracranial
hematoma,   cerebral   infarction,   and   death.   One   pain
treatment   center's   experience   suggests   that   the
best   candidates   for   deep   brain   stimulation   are
patients   with   FBS   who   are   off

narcotics and have undergone psychiatric screening. Initial pain relief is achieved in about 90% of patients and 60 to 80% obtain long term pain relief. This is often accomplished with intermittent stimulation (e.g., 3X/day), but tolerance develops in some patients. These promising results must be tempered by the serious risks involved, and this treatment should be reserved for those patients with significant disability who not do not respond to the therapies discussed above.

ADDENDUM TO CASE HISTORY:

Implantation of an epidural spinal cord stimulator yielded an estimated 80% reduction of pain. One year later, the patient continues to report similar pain relief, is off narcotic analgesics, and is working full-time in his managerial position.

4.   Generally, <u>narcotic analgesics should not be used in the treatment of benign chronic pain</u>, primarily due to the long life expectancy of the patient. The potential pain relief may not justify the major risks of narcotic therapy (i.e., drug abuse and respiratory depression), because it is generally assumed that tolerance will develop and thus limit the duration of its effectiveness. If attempted, prolonged narcotic therapy requires the maintenance of a low dose regime and the strict supervision of a single physician experienced in chronic pain treatment. <u>The infusion of morphine into the lumbar intrathecal or epidural space has been used quite effectively in the management of severe pain associated with malignant disease</u>. There is limited experience with this therapy in patients with benign chronic pain syndromes. In one small study, none of the 6 patients experienced a long term benefit, one continued to use the morphine at 1 year, reporting marginal improvement and tolerance developed in some patients. This treatment should be considered investigational.

5. <u>Neuroablative procedures carry significant risks</u> of
    producing neurological deficits and none have been
    found to offer pain relief of more than 3 to 6
    months' duration.   They do not play a role in the
    treatment of chronic pain of benign origin such as
    FBS.

REFERENCES

1. Burton CV. The failed back.   In Wilkins RH,
   Rengachary SS, eds. Neurosurgery. New York, McGraw-
   Hill, pp 2290-2292, 1985.

2. Coombs DW, Saunders RL. Intraspinal infusion of
   narcotic drugs. In Wilkins RH, Rengachary SS, eds.
   Neurysorgery. New York, McGraw-Hill, pp 2410-2414,
   1985.

3. Hendler   NH.   The   diagnosis   and   nonsurgical
   management of chronic pain. New York, Raven Press,
   1981.

4. Long   DM.   Surgical   therapy   of   chronic   pain.
   Neurosurgery 6:317-328, 1980.

5. Melzack   R,   Wall   PD.   Gate   control   theory.   In
   Wilkins RH, Rengarachary SS, eds. Neurosurgery.
   New York, McGraw-Hill, pp 2317-2319, 1985.

6. Richardson DE.   Deep   brain   stimulation   for   pain
   relief.   In   Wilkins   RH,   Rengachary   SS,   eds.
   Neurosurgery. New York, McGraw-Hill, pp 2421-
   2526, 1985.

7. Wilkinson HA.   The failed back syndrome: etiology
   and therapy. Philadelphia, Harper & Row, 1983.

SURGICAL TREATMENT OF FACIAL PAIN

CASE 27: A 70-year-old woman presented with severe facial pain. The pains lasted between 10 seconds and several minutes and were followed by a dull aching pain that persisted more than an hour. Evaluation by a neurologist revealed both normal neurological examination and CAT scan of the brain (without and with contrast). The diagnosis of trigeminal neuralgia ("tic douloureux") was made and the patient was begun on a gradually increasing dose of carbamazepine. The patient became nearly pain free, but over several months the paroxysms began to recur and increasing dosages were required for pain control. Eventually phenytoin (Dilantin) was added and initially provided a dramatic reduction of the frequency and severity of the attacks of pain. However, within 6 months, the patient was experiencing several severe episodes of pain each day and complained of nearly chronic aching of the right jaw. She was unable to chew solid food and had lost 10 kg in recent months. Neurological examination remained normal.

Neuroanatomical Clue: (See diagrams)

QUESTIONS:

1. How is trigeminal neuralgia diagnosed?

2. What are the possible etiologies of trigeminal neuralgia?

3. What are the two types of neurosurgical intervention that have proved to be the most effective in the treatment of this problem?

4. What further therapy (if any) would you recommend for the patient presented above?

5. What therapy would you recommend for a young healthy patient whose intractable pain was initially localized to the left eye and forehead?

Figure 27.1:
   (left)

Figure 27.1:
   (right)

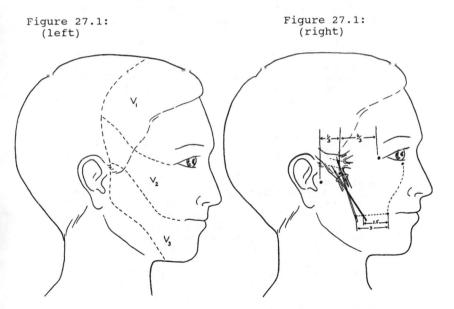

ANSWERS:

1. The key to the diagnosis of <u>trigeminal neuralgia</u>
    is the history. Generally, the neurological
    examination and tests [e.g., head computed axial
    tomography (CAT) scan] are unremarkable. The most
    important historical factors include the
    distribution of the pain and the occurrence of
    "attacks" of pain with long relatively pain-free
    intervals. The pain usually begins in the
    distribution of either the <u>second or third division
    of the trigeminal nerve</u>, and with time often
    spreads to involve the other (see Fig. 27.1). In
    some cases it begins in the distribution of the
    first division. Patients with constant trigeminal
    region pain generally demand an alternative
    diagnosis and many of them will fit into the
    syndrome of atypical facial pain. This group of
    patients generally does not benefit from the
    therapies discussed here.

2. The pathophysiological mechanism(s) underlying
    trigeminal neuralgia have not been definitively
    established, although there is an extensive
    clinical experience with this entity. As summarized
    by Wilkins (see Ref. 2), any theory of the
    mechanism for this disorder must be consistent
    with: <u>1) the paroxysmal nature of the pain</u>, with
    long pain-free intervals; 2) the frequent existence
    of <u>"trigger" stimuli</u> that are carried via large
    diameter afferents (not pain fibers) and often via
    a division of the fifth nerve other than the
    division of the pain; 3) the fact that <u>a
    small/partial lesion of the gasserian ganglion
    and/or roots often relieves the pain</u>; and 4) the
    occurrence of trigeminal neuralgia in patients with
    <u>central demyelinating disease</u> (occurs in 1% of
    patients with multiple sclerosis). These facts
    seem most consistent with a central rather than a
    peripheral nerve etiology. The paroxysms of pain
    are analogous to seizures and interestingly are
    often controlled by anticonvulsant medications
    (e.g. carbamazepine and phenytoin). It seems very
    likely that the attacks of pain may represent
    aberrant bursts of neuronal activity possibly
    initiated by innocuous input via the fifth nerve)

originating along the central tract of the fifth
nerve or at the level of its central synapses.

A variety of pathological conditions have been
implicated as possible causes for this disorder. A
large number of patients operated on for trigeminal
neuralgia have been found to have apparent
compression of the fifth nerve root entry zone at
the brain stem by a blood vessel (variously
reported to be 45 to 95% of patients). This is
presumed to increase with age secondary to the
elongation of arteries that occurs with aging and
arteriosclerosis and may be the etiology for this
disorder in many patients. An alternative
mechanism must be operating in the remaining
patients, and autopsy studies have revealed many
cases of similar apparent vascular compression in
patients that did not manifest this syndrome during
life. Nonvascular compression along the fifth
nerve occurs in some patients. Various series
report that 1-8% of patients harbor a benign
cerebellopontine angle tumor (including
meningiomas, epidermoid cysts, acoustic neuromas,
and arteriovenous malformations) and there have
been reported cases of bony compression (e.g.,
secondary to Paget's disease). Unlike most
patients with trigeminal neuralgia, these patients
often have symptoms and/or signs of cranial nerve
deficits. Other possible causes include peripheral
fifth nerve injury (e.g., a dental procedure) or
multiple sclerosis, while some patients have no
apparent pathology.

3. Destructive lesions and decompressive procedures
    represent the two general types of neurosurgical
    intervention that have proved to be the most
    effective in the treatment of medically refractory
    trigeminal neuralgia. Currently the destructive
    lesions are made almost exclusively by percutaneous
    approach to the gasserian ganglion (via radio-
    frequency thermocoagulation and/or glycerol
    injection). This procedure utilizes skull x-ray
    landmarks to introduce a long thin needle through
    the cheek to the area of the gasserian ganglion by
    penetrating the foramen ovale. An electrode passed
    through the needle is stimulated to determine the

location of the tip (first, second, or third division). Once precise location is achieved (either to the distribution of the pain or the trigger stimulus), current is applied to heat the tip in order to create a precise and partial lesion of the gasserian ganglion. When the tip lays in the cerebrospinal fluid (CSF) bathing the gasserian ganglion, some surgeons instill glycerol (either in addition to or in place of heat) to generate a partial lesion. This procedure can generally be done on an out-patient basis in a same-day surgery setting. Several large series of patients have been reported with no mortality. Transient herpetic eruptions following the procedure are relatively common. The rare serious morbidity following thermocoagulation has included denervation induced severely painful paresthesias or dysesthesias (anesthesia dolorosa) and neurolytic keratitis (with potential blindness), each with a less than 1% incidence. Up to 5% have complained of annoying paresthesias or dysesthesias.

Puncture of the internal carotid artery has occurred, but this is generally well tolerated. Relief of pain in a series of 800 patients reported by Nugent (see Ref. 2) was rated as excellent in 62%, good in 25%, fair in 7%, and poor in 6%, with recurrent pain requiring a second procedure in 23%. A large series of glycerol lesioned patients has been reported with no serious complications. In this group, 66% were pain free at follow-up (13% having required a second injection) and 19% had good relief with medication. Of the 15% with inadequate relief, 1/3 were relieved by thermocoagulation. Another series reported only 4% with inadequate relief.

Exploration of the fifth nerve and its root entry zone, with the objective of alleviating any vascular compression (if present), has developed as an alternative effective treatment of trigeminal neuralgia (termed microvascular decompression or MVD). MVD is aimed at the proposed etiology of this syndrome, as opposed to the empiric symptomatically oriented procedure discussed above.

MVD involves a retromastoid craniectomy (or craniotomy) for an infratentorial exposure of the fifth nerve. Treatment involves the moving or cushioning of any compressing arteries and the coagulation and removal of any compressing veins. In a series of 410 patients reported by Jannetta (Ref. 2), vascular compression was identified in 392 (242 arterial, 96 arteriovenous, 54 venous), a mass lesion in 17, and no lesion in two patients. To summarize the results, MVD yielded pain relief in 80% of patients, with repeated operation able to increase this to 84%. After MVD, an additional 4% responded to thermocoagulation and 9% to medication. Of the remainder, 2% had reduced pain and 1% had severe pain. This group included 2 postoperative deaths (0.5%) and serious complications occurred in a total of 15% (including permanent cranial nerve deficits, transient aseptic meningitis, intracranial hematoma, bacterial meningitis, infarction, pneumonia, CSF rhinorrhea and pulmonary embolus). A subsequent 400 patients have been reported with no mortality, but with an increased frequency of transient aseptic meningitis (30 versus 5%). Of interest is the fact that pain relief was obtained in only 43% of patients who had undergone a prior destructive lesion.

4. This patient would be an ideal candidate for a percutaneous lesion directed at the third division of the fifth nerve. This is a simple, safe and effective procedure that can be accomplished without the risk of general anesthesia in this patient with a history of myocardial infarction. If CSF flow is obtained from the needle, glycerol (with less morbidity, but also possibly less efficacy than thermocoagulation) might be the method of choice for lesioning, while thermocoagulation remains as arguably an equally good alternative.

CASE HISTORY ADDENDUM:

This patient underwent a percutaneous gasserian ganglion lesion as an outpatient under local anesthesia. A good flow of CSF was obtained on needle placement and stimulation elicited a tingling of the right lower lip.   A partial lesion was made by thermocoagulation and a small amount of glycerol was injected after determining that pinprick and corneal sensation were still present.   Following the procedure the patient did have hypesthesia.   Phenytoin was discontinued and the patient returned home on a tapering schedule of carbamezepine.   At follow-up 1 year later the patient was off medications and pain free.

5.   This can be a more complex decision than for the elderly patient described above.   Since this patient has a long life expectancy, no increased general anesthesia risks, and pain involving the ophthalmic division of the fifth nerve (increasing the risk of neurolytic keratitis with a ganglion lesion), he would be an ideal candidate for MVD (with partial lesioning intraoperatively if no compression is found).   Alternatively, many patients with forehead pain respond to lesions of the supraorbital nerve at its exit from the orbit. This might be tried prior to proceeding with an operation, although there is some risk of subsequent painful paresthesias or dysesthesias with this treatment.   It is of utmost importance, however, that the decision regarding therapy in this or any case is a joint decision between the patient and his physician.   In each case the alternatives are explained and the patient decides what he or she feels is best.

REFERENCES

1. Hassler R, Walker AE, eds. Trigeminal neuralgia: pathogenesis and pathophysiology. Stuttgart, Thieme, 1970.

2. Wilkins RH, Nugent GR, Lunsford LD, Jannetta PJ. Trigeminal Neuralgia. In Wilkins RH, Rengachary SS, eds. Neurosurgery. New York, McGraw-Hill, pp 2337-2363, 1985.

WOMAN WITH POSTERIOR FOSSA LESION

CASE 28: A 45-year-old woman presented with nausea, vomiting, severe headache, and inability to stand. Neurological evaluation revealed bilateral papilledema, a right VIth and VIIth nerve palsy, left hemiparesis, and wide based ataxic gait with frequent falling to her right side. These symptoms had been gradually worsening over the 7 days prior to admission. Her past history was significant for a modified radical mastectomy of the left breast over 4 years ago at which time no evidence of lymph node involvement or other spread of the cancer was detected. She had not received radiation or chemotherapy at that time and current checkups revealed no evidence of recurrence.

Clue:

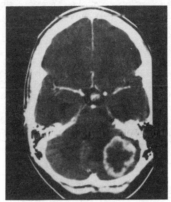

Figure 28.1   Computed tomography (CT) scan of head

QUESTIONS:

1. What is the diagnosis? Is the time course typical?

2. By what routes do metastatic lesions reach the central nervous system?

3. What are the principles of management in such cases?

4. Are other investigations necessary?

5. What is the expected outcome?

ANSWERS:

1. The most likely diagnosis given the history of
    breast cancer in this patient harboring an
    enhancing mass in the posterior fossa is a
    <u>metastasis</u>. The history of a latent metastasis in
    a patient with either breast cancer or a melanoma
    is not uncommon, even with the absence of any known
    recurrence from the primary tumor. Breast cancer
    metastasis usually results in a solitary brain
    lesion that frequently can be completely excised
    from the surrounding brain tissue. Because patients
    with breast cancer have an increased incidence of
    meningioma, this lesion should be kept in the
    differential diagnosis.

2. The great majority of lesions reach the central
    nervous system (CNS) by <u>hematogenous spread</u> and
    therefore are distributed according to the arterial
    anatomy and blood supply of the brain. Two other
    routes are direct spread from contiguous soft
    tissue and bony structures surrounding the brain
    and skull or by venous spread thru Batson's spinal
    epidural venous plexus. As the brain has no
    lymphatic system, spread cannot occur along this
    route.

3. The treatment of a solitary intracranial metastasis
    is a function of many factors including the
    specific type and grade of tumor, the sensitivity
    of the tumor to radiation or chemotherapy, the time
    interval from diagnosis of the primary cancer to
    the appearance of the metastasis, the size and
    location of tumor in the central nervous system,
    the clinical condition and age of the patient, and
    the degree of dissemination of the primary cancer.
    Most patients who harbor an intracranial metastasis
    have widely disseminated cancer and the treatment
    is solely palliative and consists of steroids and
    possible radiation or chemotherapy. In this case,
    however, the patient is generally healthy without
    overt evidence of disseminated cancer and the
    metastasis is in a location (posterior fossa) where
    nonsurgical therapy would result in the rapid
    demise of this patient. Surgical removal of this
    tumor will result in a conformation of the
    diagnosis, alleviate the symptoms of posterior

fossa compression and hydrocephalus, and allow
sufficient time for further evaluation and therapy
in this patient.

4. After surgical removal or decompression of this
    tumor, the patient should be evaluated for the
    presence of other metastasis as this will greatly
    influence treatment and outcome in this case. In
    addition to obtaining bone scans, CT of the
    abdomen, and a repeat mammography, the patient
    should have a lumbar puncture with cytological
    analysis of the cerebrospinal   fluid (CSF). Th
    last test is important as breast cancer metastasis
    to the CNS can have an associated carcinomatous
    meningitis.

5. The outcome in the majority of patients with brain
    metastasis is poor. Most patients at the time of
    central nervous system involvement have widely
    disseminated disease and have suffered the
    debilitating effects of systemic cancer treatments
    on the bone marrow, lungs, and cardiovascular
    system. The median survival is usually less than 9
    months but in selected patients with single lesions
    and no evidence of cancer elsewhere, surgical
    excision with adjuvant therapy may result in the
    possibility of a cure or long term remission.

PEARLS:

1. The central nervous system is a frequent site for
    metastasis from primary tumors. Autopsy studies
    reveal 12-35% of patients with cancer will have CNS
    involvement at the time of death and half of all
    brain tumors diagnosed are secondary to metastasis.

2. The most frequent cancers to involve the CNS are
    lung, breast, gastrointestinal, melanoma, and
    lymphoma.

3. In 9% of cases, the brain represents the only site
    of metastasis of the cancer.

4. Forty to forty-five percent of metastasis are
    solitary and most involve the cerebral hemispheres
    (80%) with less frequent involvement of cerebellum
    (16%) and brain stem (4%).

5.   Cerebral hemorrhage secondary to a brain metastasis usually is seen with renal cell cancer, choriocarcinoma, and melanoma.

6.   Spread to the leptomeninges resulting in <u>carcinomatous meningitis</u> is usually associated with the following cancers: breast, lung, melanoma, or lymphoma.

7.   In children, metastatic involvement is less common and is seen only in 6% of cases. The tumors involved are neuroblastoma, rhabdomyosarcoma, and Wilms' tumor.

8.   Single metastasis is more common in breast, renal, and ovarian cancer where multiple metastases are more common in lung, melanoma, and colonic metastasis.

PITFALLS:

1.   The differential diagnosis of an intracerebral mass in a cancer patient should include the possibility of a brain abscess (especially in immunosuppressed patients), intracerebral hematoma (due to thrombocytopenia), or other primary brain tumors (meningiomas in breast/prostate cancer).

2.   Size of a metastasis is a poor indication of the degree of edema these lesions cause, especially in white matter where a small metastatic deposit may induce widespread cerebral edema.

REFERENCES

1. Galicich JH, Sundaresan N, Arbit E, Passe S: Surgical treatment of single brain metastasis: factors associated with survival. Cancer 45:391-386, 1980.

2. Galicich JH, Sundaresan N, Thaler HT: Surgical treatment of single brain metastasis: evaluation of results by computerized tomography scan. J Neurosurg 53:63-70, 1980.

3. Lokich JJ: Management of cerebral metastasis. JAMA 234:748-751, 1975.

4. Patchell RA: Single brain matastasis: surgery plus radiation or radiation alone. Neurology 36(4):447-453, 1986.

5. Pechoua-Peteroua V: CT findings in cerebral metastasis. Neuroradiology 28(3):254-258, 1986.

6. Posner JB, Chernik NL: Intracranial metastasis from systemic cancer. Adv Neurol 19:579-592, 1978.

7. Sarma DP: Long-term survival after brain metastasis from lung cancer. Cancer 58 (6): 1366-1370, 1986.

8. Snee MP: Brain metastases from carcinoma of the breast: a review of 90 cases. Clin Radiol 36 (4):365-367, 1985.

9. Wilson CB: Brain metastases: basis for surgical selection. Int J Radiat Oncol Biol Phys 2:169-172, 1977.

CASE 29: A 41-year-old man with a 3-week history of low back pain was referred by his internist with a three week history of low back pain. The patient stated that the pain was first noticed 1 day after lifting heavy furniture. A week prior to presentation the pain began to radiate to the left lower extremity. Specifically, the patient stated that the pain went down the posterior aspect of the left thigh into the lateral aspect of the leg and medially across the dorsum of the foot to the great toe. There was no reported weakness in the lower extremities and no change in the patient's bowel, bladder, or sexual function. He reported no overt sensory loss but stated that he occasionally had "pins and needles" sensations in the lateral aspect of his left leg and the left great toe.

On physical examination the patient appeared in no distress.

There was no spinal or paraspinal tenderness. Straight leg raising was positive on the left at 60 degrees. Reverse straight leg raising was negative.

Neurological motor examination showed a mild decrease in the strength of great toe extension on the left. There was no demonstrable sensory defect. Deep tendon reflexes were normally active and symmetrical.

Plain anteroposterior (AP) and lateral x-rays of the lumbar spine were normal.

Clue: Figure 29.1: Schematic drawing of the lumbosacral spine and nerve roots

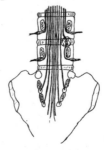

QUESTIONS:

1. What is your differential diagnosis at this point?
   Can you localize the pathology in the neuroaxis?

2. Do you want any additional radiographic
   examinations?

3. Discuss the significance of a positive crossed
   straight leg raising sign in this disease process.

4. Most lumbar intervertebral discs herniate laterally.
   Discuss the findings which can occur if a lumbar
   disc herniates centrally.

5. What are the indications for surgical treatment of
   lumbar disc herniation?

6. Is surgery for lumbar disc herniation more effective
   than conservative management with bed rest?

7. Is there a role for chymopapain disc injection in
   the treatment of a herniated nucleus pulposus?

ANSWERS:

1. Low back pain can be caused by a variety of disorders including bony and muscular disorders and even tumors. Lumbar disc herniation (actually herniation of the nucleus pulposus through the annulus of the disc), however, is one of the most common causes of low back pain. When pain radiates to the lower extremities (sciatica) this is indicative of nerve root compression or irritation, often from a herniated disc. To localize the exact root involved certain elements of the history and physical must be considered. The pattern of pain can be suggestive of a specific nerve root but is not always reliable. Motor, sensor, and reflex findings on physical examination must be considered together when attempting to localize a radiculopathy. Table 29.1 summarizes the clinical findings associated with lesions of the various lumbar roots.

    Table 29.1:

Disc Space	L3-4	L4-5	L5-S1
Root involved	L4	L5	S1
Weakness	Quadriceps	Anterior tibial, Extensor Hallucis Longus	Gastroc-nemius
Sensory loss	Anterior thigh	Great toe, lateral leg	Lateral foot
Reflex loss	Knee jerk	Posterior tibial	Ankle jerk

    When a lumbar intervertebral disc herniates it usually causes compression of the next lower nerve root. That is to say if the L4-5 disc herniates, nerve compression if present would most likely involve the L5 root.

The most common lumbar disc to herniate is L4-5
followed by L5-S1.   In this patient we see clinical
evidence of left L5 nerve root compression.   Thus
we suspect a herniated disc at the L4-L5 level
lateralizing to the left.

2.   Plain x-rays of the spine are of limited usefulness
in   the   evaluation   of   patients   with   acutely
herniated discs.   They can show degenerative bony
changes and spondylolisthesis which may also give
rise to low back pain, but plain x-rays cannot
confirm or exclude the presence of a herniated
disc.   Often, a herniated disc is suggested by a
decrease in the height of the disc space.

Myelography has traditionally been the procedure
of choice in the evaluation of suspected herniated
discs.   It has a sensitivity of approximately 75%
and   a   specificity   of   around   90%.   Currently,
computed tomography (CT) and magnetic resonance
imaging (MRI) scanning are often used as the first
radiological test in the evaluation of suspected
disc herniation.   They have the advantage of being
noninvasive, and MRI scanning can be done in the
sagittal plane thus demonstrating the relationship
of the disc to the thecal sac quite clearly.
Surgery   is   being   performed   with   increasing
frequency on the basis of CT and MRI scans alone,
however,   myelography   is   still   commonly   used
especially when CT or MRI fails to clearly
demonstrate a lesion.

In   this   patient   lumbar   CT   scanning   and
myelography were performed.   These are shown in
Figures 29.2 and 29.3, respectively.

Figure 29.2:   CT scan of lumbar spine

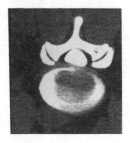

Figure 29.3:   Lumbar myelogram

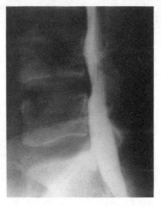

3.   A <u>positive straight leg raising</u> sign in the
     clinical setting consistent with lumbar disc
     herniation confirms the diagnosis in >60% of cases.
     The crossed straight leg raising sign is the
     production of pain in the symptomatic extremity
     when the contralateral extremity is passively
     raised with the patient supine and the knee
     straight. This is confirmatory of a herniated
     lumbar disc in >95% of cases.

4.   Should lumbar disc herniation occur centrally, the
     symptoms and signs are classically those of <u>cauda
     equina compression</u>. These include lower extremity
     weakness, urinary retention, constipation, sacral
     anesthesia, and decreased anal sphincter tone.
     Central lumbar disc herniation with neurological
     symptoms is a surgical emergency and immediate
     decompression should be provided.

5.   Surgery on the lumbar spine is the most frequent
     type of surgery performed by neurosurgeons in the
     United States. In the treatment of acute herniated
     lumbar disc a partial laminectomy with foramenotomy
     is usually performed with removal of as much disc
     material as possible.

The decision to operate of course depends on the clinical situation and radiographic findings. Most surgeons feel that operation is not usually indicated for low back pain alone without radiculopathy unless associated with an anatomically appropriate neurological deficit. <u>When radicular pain is associated with motor weakness in the appropriate neurological distribution operation is indicated</u>. At this point low back pain may or may not be present. In patients with sciatica without neurological findings a 2-week trial of bed rest, should be the first line of treatment. If satisfactory results are not obtained after an adequate trial of bed rest then operation may be considered.

6.   There are numerous studies describing the natural history of low back pain with and without lumbar radiculopathy. In addition there are long-term post-operative studies of patients surgically treated for herniated lumbar discs. However, there is only 1 study which compared surgical to non-surgical treatment of herniated lumbar discs in a prospective randomized manner. In this study the surgical group had a statistically significant better outcome at the end of 1 year than the conservatively managed group. By 4 and 10 years the surgical group still showed better results but the difference was no longer statistically significant.

     There are no infallible preoperative predictors of success or failure in lumbar disc surgery, but factors which indicate the presence of an acutely herniated disc in the absence of other spinal pathology (especially significant degenerative disease) often correlate with a good outcome. Factors correlating with a better outcome include: age <45 years, absence of significant osteophyte formation on lumbar spine x-ray, nonsedentary lifestyle, and absence of secondary gain from the disability (such as compensatory claims).

7.   <u>Chymopapain</u> is a proteolytic enzyme which breaks down mucopolysaccharides present in the nucleus pulposus. It is quite toxic when given

systemically or intrathecally. When injected into the disc space chymopapain hydrolyzes a portion of the mucopolysaccharides thus possibly decreasing the size of the nucleus and alleviating symptoms.

Although many patients have been treated with chymopapain, the completed results of prospective controlled studies are not yet available. It appears that about 60-70% of patients treated with intradiscal chymopapain injection experience some benefit whereas placebo is effective in about 50%. By comparison conservative management with best rest is effective also in 60-70% of patients and surgery is effective in more than 85%. Thus the initial enthusiasm for chymopapain treatment has not been widely sustained.

PEARLS:

1.   Approximately <u>80% of people experience significant low back pain</u> at sometime in their lives.

2.   About 35% of these individuals will develop sciatica.

3.   Low back pain usually precedes the development of sciatica by 6-10 years.

4.   The crossed straight leg-raising sign when present indicates a herniated disc >95% of the time.

5.   <u>Most disc disease presents between the ages of 40-60 years</u>. It is rare before the age of 25 or after the age of 60.

6.   Eighty percent of disc disease occurs in men.

PITFALLS:

1.   In 6% of patients there occurs an anatomical variant in which <u>there may be only 4 lumbar vertebral bodies (sacralized lumbar spine) or 6 lumbar vertebral bodies (lumberized spine)</u>. This anomaly will obviously affect the usual disc level and its associated symptoms and signs.

2. Although rare, <u>approximately 5% of lumbar discs
    occur at L1, L2, or L3</u>. These discs frequently
    present with symptoms of cauda equina compression.

3. <u>Myelography may miss lateral or foraminal disc</u>
    extrusions. CT scans or MRI will demonstrate these
    lateral fragments well.

REFERENCES

1. Weber H: Lumbar disc herniation: a controlled,
   prospective study with ten years of observation.
   Spine 8:131-140, 1983.

2. Lewis PJ, Weir BKA, Broad RW, Grace MG: Long term
   prospective study of lumbosacral discectomy. J
   Neurosurg 67:49-53, 1987.

3. Hudgins WR: The predictive value of myelography in
   the diagnosis of ruptured lumbar discs. J Neurosurg
   32:152-162, 1970.

4. Murphy F: Experience with lumbar disc surgery.
   Clinical Neurosurgery 20.1 8, 1973.

5. Watts C: Current status of chymopapain. In Hardy RW,
   ed. Lumbar disc disease. New York, Raven Press,
   1982, pp 157-164.

6. Hudgins WR: The crossed-straight-leg-raising test.
   N Engl J Med 297:1127, 1977.

SEVERAL-YEAR HISTORY OF LOW BACK AND LEFT LEG PAIN WITH ASSOCIATED LEFT LEG WEAKNESS AND DIFFICULTY WITH MICTURITION

CASE 30: A 35-year-old woman presented with a 6-year history of low back pain. Four years ago the patient noted radiation of her pain into the left anterior thigh and painful dysesthesias in the same distribution. One year ago the patient began to have difficulties with her gait particularly with climbing stairs. In the past 6 months she noted difficulties with bladder function describing an inability to sense bladder fullness and intermittent dribbling incontinence.

The admission examination was notable for weakness and atrophy of the left quadriceps muscle. The left patellar reflex was absent and the left achilles reflex was hypoactive. There was decreased light touch and pain sensation in the left L3 and L4 dermatome as well as some decrease in perineal sensation on the left. Urodynamic studies revealed incomplete lower motor neuron dysfunction of the bladder.

Iohexal myelography revealed an intradural mass at the L2 vertebral level. The patient underwent operative exploration via a posterior laminectomy. A well encapsulated tumor was encountered arising from the L3 dorsal root. A complete removal of the tumor was accomplished although most of the left L3 dorsal root was sacrificed. Postoperatively the pain completely resolved and bladder function returned to normal. The left quadriceps remains weak and there is numbness in the L3 dermatome on the left. Pathological examination of the tumor revealed a neurofibroma.

CLUE: Radicular pain and dysfunction in the leg is most frequently caused by disc herniation. About 90-95% of all lumbar disc herniations occur at the L4-L5 or L5-S1 levels. Patients presenting with radicular dysfunction in roots other than L5 or S1 should be suspected of harboring a tumor of the cauda equina.

QUESTIONS:

1. Describe the clinical features and common causes of the cauda equina syndrome.

2. What features in the history and examination of this patient were helpful in suggesting the correct preoperative diagnosis?

3. Which radiological procedures should be obtained preoperatively?

4. What is the treatment of these tumors?

ANSWERS:

1. The <u>cauda equina syndrome</u> is a general term used to describe a variable degree of dysfunction of any combination of roots of the cauda equina. Because the cauda equina is composed of most of the lumbar and all of the sacral roots, the clinical features of this syndrome include <u>pain, weakness, and sensory loss in one or both legs as well as disturbances of bowel and bladder</u> function and decreased perineal sensation.

    The most common <u>causes of the cauda equina syndrome include tumors and lumbar stenosis</u>. Herniated discs, particularly if the herniations are central, may also produce this syndrome. Neurofibromas arising from the nerve roots of the cauda equina, and filum terminale ependymomas are the most common tumors in this region. Meningiomas and metastatic tumors are less frequently encountered. In the pediatric population, inclusion tumors such as dermoids, lipomas, and teratomas, which are associated with the occult dysraphic states, may also produce cauda equina compression.

2. <u>Spinal neurofibromas</u> usually arise from a dorsal sensory root. Because they are slow growing tumors signs of spinal cord or nerve root compression occur late in the clinical course of these patients. Frequently, pain in the radicular distribution of the nerve root origin of the tumor will be the earliest symptom produced by a spinal neurofibroma. In this patient the early appearance of pain radiating to the left anterior thigh and followed later by weakness in the left quadriceps muscle suggested the correct diagnosis of neurofibroma arising from the left L3 nerve root.

3. <u>Myelography and postmyelography computerized tomography</u> (CT) are the most useful radiological studies to be obtained preoperatively. Myelography identifies the rostral-caudal extent of the tumor and will usually disclose whether the tumor is predominantly intra- or extradural. The performance of post myelography CT better defines the relationship of the tumor to the thecal sac and

spinal cord. Extraspinal extension through an enlarged intervertebral foramen will also be visualized with CT.

Magnetic resonance imaging (MRI) has developed into a particularly sensitive and useful test employed in the imaging of spinal tumors. The noninvasive nature of MRI makes it an ideal screening procedure and, in some institutions, it has replaced myelography and CT in the radiological evaluation of spinal tumors.

4. The treatment of spinal neurofibromas is surgical extirpation. These are benign well encapsulated tumors which are moderately vascular. Total excision is usually possible although larger tumors with extraspinal extension may require a staged or combined anterior and posterior approach.

PEARLS:

1. Neurofibromas are the most common intradural extramedullary spinal tumor. They occur anywhere along the spinal axis where they usually arise from a dorsal root. About 20% of spinal neurofibromas arise from the roots of the cauda equina. The majority of these tumors are entirely intradural but about 15-20% have both intra and extradural components. In about 10% of patients an extradural component extends through an intervertebral foramen and assumes a dumbbell shape with both intraspinal and paraspinal growth.

2. There is much more variation and overlap in the motor innervation as compared to the rather limited overlap in the sensory dermatomes in the leg. Therefore, the sensory examination of the leg will more accurately identify the affected spinal nerves. This situation is reversed in the arm where motor deficits more accurately define the site of the lesion.

PITFALLS:

1. The average duration of symptoms preceding diagnosis in patients with neurofibromas of the cauda equina is about 5 years.

    This reflects the slow growth rate of these tumors and, because these tumors arise below the termination of the spinal cord, compression of the spinal cord does not usually occur.

    Failure to appreciate early or subtle signs, particularly the appearance of radicular pain, will delay diagnosis. This delay allows these tumors to attain a large size which makes surgery much more difficult and frequently results in incomplete removal.

REFERENCES

1. Fearnside MR, Adams CBT: Tumors of the cauda equina. J Neurol Neurosurg Psych 41:24-31, 1978.

2. Norstrom CW, Kernohan JW, Love JG: One hundred primary caudal tumors. JAMA 178:93-99, 1961.

3. Rubinstein LJ: The malformative central nervous system lesions in the central and peripheral forms of neurofibromatosis. A neuropathological study of 22 cases. Ann NY Acad Sci 486:14-29, 1986.

4. Scotti G, Scialfa G, Colombo N, et al: Magnetic resonance diagnosis of intramedullary tumors of the spinal cord. Neuroradiology 29(2):130-135, 1987.

5. Solomon RA, Handler MS, Sedilli RV, et al: Intramedullary melanotic schwannoma of the cervicomedullary junction. Neurosurgery 20(1):36-38, 1987.

10-TEN-MONTH OLD WITH "FUNNY HEAD"

CASE 31: A mother brings her 10-month-old child to the hospital. Her mother-in-law thinks that the child's head looks "funny." The child appears to be quite happy. He has met all of his milestones. On examination, the only abnormality is that his forehead above his left eye appears to be flat. The anterior fontanelle is not closed but there is a slight ridge palpable above the left forehead.

CLUE: Harlequin sign on anteroposterior (AP) skull

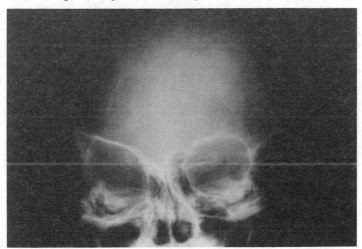

Figure 31.1

1. What is the diagnosis in this case and what is the pathogenesis of this problem?

2. How would you investigate it?

3. Would you do anything?

4. What would you do?

5. When would you do it?

ANSWERS:

1. <u>The child has unilateral coronal synostosis i.e.
   Plagiocephaly</u>. Craniosynostosis was described by
   Virchow in 1851 as craniostenosis. It may be
   thought of as primary, reflecting premature closure
   of cranial sutures because of an abnormality of the
   development of the skull, and as secondary, due to
   an abnormality of the underlying brain. Primary
   synostosis occurs in approximately .05% of live
   births. It can occur at any suture in the skull
   and the etiology is unknown. The bones of the
   calvarium develop in membrane from the 6th week of
   intrauterine life; the bones of the base of the
   skull develop in cartilage. One theory proposes
   that the bones of the base of the skull exert an
   influence over the calvarial bones via dural struts
   and that the primary abnormality is in the basal
   bones. Other explanations include abnormal fetal
   position, infection in utero, genetic determinants,
   and metabolic derangements, especially rickets.

   <u>The metopic suture closes before birth</u> (a
   midline frontal suture between the two halves of
   the frontal bone), the <u>posterior fontanelle at 3
   months, the anterior fontanelle at 18 months and
   after age 12 an increase in intracranial pressure
   will not result in increased skull size</u>. Virchow's
   law states that growth of the skull takes place at
   right angles to the sutures; if a suture closes
   prematurely, the skull and brain grow parallel to
   the suture.

   Sagittal synostosis thus causes the skull to
   grow long, like a boat: <u>scaphocephaly</u>. Bilateral
   coronal synostosis causes the skull to grow
   laterally giving a broad shallow skull:
   <u>brachycephaly</u>. Unilateral coronal synostosis
   causes an uneven forehead: <u>Plagiocephaly</u>. Lambdoid
   synostosis causes flattening of the base of the
   skull (this is rare): <u>posterior plagiocephaly</u>.
   Premature closure of the metopic suture causes
   <u>trigonocephaly</u>, with a ridge in the middle of the
   forehead. Closure of all of the sutures results in
   a high pointed head: <u>oxycephaly</u>. Sagittal
   synostosis is probably the most common single

suture abnormality. Bilateral coronal synostosis
is commonly associated with craniofacial
abnormalities. Any combination may occur.

2. The first step is plain x-ray. This should be done
    in all cases and in the case of coronal synostosis
    the characteristic "Harlequin Eye" sign may be seen
    (see Fig. 31.1). Computed tomography (CT) should
    be done where possible, but not necessarily so for
    simple sagittal synostosis. In some centers, a 3-
    dimensional CT reconstruction of the skull is
    available which gives a spectacular image of the
    lesion.

3. Most surgery for synostosis is done for cosmetic
    reasons. There is some evidence that even in
    single suture synostosis there is an increase in
    intracranial pressure. However, in most such cases,
    intellectual development is normal if no
    reconstruction is attempted. If more than one
    suture is involved, there is a greater chance of
    neurological impairment, specifically visual, motor,
    and cognitive problems. These cases should be
    reconstructed. If it is available with low
    morbidity and minimal mortality, surgery should be
    offered for single suture synostosis. A normal
    brain in an abnormally shaped head is a recipe for
    unhappiness.

4. The problem with this child is related to the
    sphenorbital bone system and to correct it, the
    superior margin of the orbital must be advanced,
    requiring a combined intracranial and facial
    approach. For bilateral coronal synostosis
    associated with Crouzon's syndrome and other
    craniofacial abnormalities, this must be done on
    both sides.

    The first efforts at craniectomy for this
condition involved simply removing the suture. The
problem with this was rapid reclosure.
Consequently polyethylene and other barrier
materials were used to prevent this, as was
Zenker's solution. The former have been largely
abandoned; the latter has been shown to be harmful.
A more aggressive approach involved total

craniectomy, allowing the dura to adopt its own spherical shape and thus order bone growth. Sagittal synostosis is now treated with wide craniectomy of the involved suture, with or without dividing the adjacent parietal bones into small pieces (morcellation). All were made more reasonable with better craniotomes. This child had a combined neurosurgical plastic procedure using a bifrontal incision with advancement of the left superior orbital margin. He had a smooth perioperative course and a good result. This abnormality tends to worsen as the child ages if it is not reconstructed.

5.   The earlier the better from a cosmetic point of view, but between the 6th month and the first birthday is optimal.

PEARLS AND PITFALLS:

1.   Thirty percent of patients with unilateral coronal synostosis and 60% with bilateral coronal synostosis have associated abnormalities as do a smaller number with sagittal synostosis. Craniofacial syndromes should be sought as should neurological (hydrocephalus, Chiari malformation, spina bifida, agenesis of the corpus callosum, holoprosencephaly and nonneurological problems (syndactyly, cleft lip and palate, and congenital heart disease).

2.   Postional molding of the skull may occur in infants who spend long periods of time lying on the backs of their heads such as neonates that require prolonged intensive care unit (ICU). Usually the posterior aspect of the skull becomes flatted and this may be mistaken for lambdoid synostosis.

3.   A common source of postoperative morbidity in young children undergoing correction of a cranial synostosis is related to the need for postoperative transfusions. As the circulating blood volume of children is small (approximately 80 ml/kg) hemostasis during surgery is required to reduce the need for postoperative blood replacement.

4. The first description of craniosynostosis in
    Western literature is in Homer's Iliad. In the
    Catalogue of the Ships, Thersites is described as a
    quarrelsome fellow but a powerful orator:

    > He was indeed the ugliest man who went to Troy.
    > Bowlegged, lame, his shoulders met across his
    > chest and on top it all, he had a pointed head
    > with short and stubbly hair.

    This is a classic description of rickets with
    oxycephaly. Of interest is the fact that he must
    have had relatively normal mental development. The
    basis of craniosynostosis in metabolic disorders is
    not known.

REFERENCES

1. Homer: Iliados B 215-220

2. Virchow R: Ueber der Cretinismus namentlich in
   Franken und ueber pathologisch Schadelformen. Verh
   Phys-Med Gles Wurzburg 2:230, 1851.

3. Lane LC: Iioneer craniectomy for relief of mental
   imbecility due to premature sutural closure and
   microcephalus. JAMA 18:49-50, 1892.

4. Venes JL, Bordi A: Proposed role of the
   orbitosphenoid in craniofacial dyostosis. Concepts
   Pediatr Neurosurg 5:126-135, 1985.

5. Hoffman H: The scientific basis of clinical
   practice. In Crockard A, Hayward R, Hoff J, eds:
   Neurosurgery. Oxford, Blackwell, 1985, pp 55-65.

6. Kee DB, O'Brien MS. Surgical management of
   craniosynostosis. Contemp Neurosurg 7:9-10, 1985.

RAPID ONSET OF HEMIPLEGIA WITH ACUTE INTRACEREBRAL HEMORRHAGE

CASE 32: The patient is a 45-year-old moderately obese woman healthy except for a 5 year history of poorly controlled hypertension. On the day of admission, after completing her usual 1 mile bicycle ride, she suddenly developed a generalized headache with nausea and vomiting. She then developed weakness affecting her entire left side, which rapidly progressed over several minutes to a complete hemiplegia. In addition, she was also noted to have slurred speech and to become progressively less responsive over the half hour it took to transport her to the emergency room.

On admission her blood pressure was 180/110, and she was unresponsive to verbal commands. Her cranial nerve examination revealed a marked right gaze preference and a poorly reactive right pupil. She had a flaccid left hemiplegia with ankle clonus and a positive Babinski sign on the left side.

An emergency computed tomography (CT) scan revealed a large hyperdense mass, consistent with an acute bleed, centered about the right putamen. This mass extended medially up to and included the internal capsule and extended laterally as far as the insula. Blood was present throughout the ventricular system. There was a significant right to left shift of the midline. An emergency angiogram showed no vascular anomalies.

CLUE: The location of the acute intracerebral hemorrhage (ICH) combined with the patient's history of poorly controlled hypertension suggests the likely diagnosis (see P. 188).

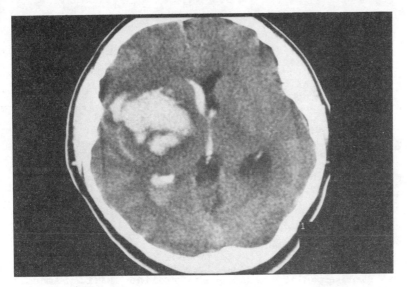

Figure 32.1

QUESTIONS:

1. What clinical features characterize the onset of an acute ICH? Which symptoms are associated with an acute bleed in this particular location?

2. What are the associated risk factors?

3. What are the most frequently involved structures?

4. What is the underlying pathophysiology of ICH?

5. What is the prognosis of recovering from such a catastrophic event? What medical or surgical types of intervention can improve the outcome?

ANSWERS:

1. Acute ICH often occurs during or following
    physicalexertion. In approximately 2/3 of these
    cases   there   is   progressive   neurological
    deterioration while in 1/3 maximal deficits are
    present at the outset.   A reduction in level of
    consciousness occurs about 60% of the time with 2/3
    of these patients progressing to coma.   Headache
    and nausea with vomiting occur in about 20 to 40%
    of these cases.   These symptoms arise from the
    increased   intracranial   pressure   caused   by   the
    bleed.   Seizures at the onset are less common,
    occurring about 7 to 14% of the time.   Other
    symptoms and signs depend on the specific location
    and size of the blood clot. The characteristics of
    a basal ganglia, usually putaminal, hemorrhage are
    a contralateral motor deficit and ipsilateral gaze
    preference   along   with   sensory,   visual,   and
    behavioral changes.   The pupillary changes seen in
    this case reflect the impending temporal lobe uncal
    herniation resulting from the combined increased
    intracranial pressure and midline shift.   Aphasic
    symptoms may also be present when the dominant
    hemisphere is involved.

2. Hypertension is found in 70 to 90% of the cases of
    ICH.   This is reflected in its higher incidence
    among black people. Two-thirds of the cases of ICH
    occur between the ages of 45 to 75 years old with
    men having a 5 to 20% higher incidence as compared
    to women.   People having a coagulopathy are at
    increased risk for an ICH as are patients on
    anticoagulation   medicine,   especially   Coumadin.
    Thrombocytopenia with a platelet count of less than
    20,000, liver disease, leukemia, and drugs such as
    amphetamine all increase the risk of suffering an
    ICH.

3. ICH occurs in the vascular territory of the small
    perforating arteries such as the lenticulostriates
    of the basal ganglia, thalamoperforators of the
    diencephalon, and basilar paramedian branches of
    the pons.   Therefore most occur within the deep
    structures   of   the   cerebral   hemispheres.   The
    following is a list of structures and their
    frequency of involvement: putamen, 30 to 50%,

subcortical white matter, 30%; cerebellum, 16%; thalamus, 10 to 15%; and pons 5 to 12%.

4. ICHs comprise approximately 10% of all strokes. As discussed above they result from an arterial bleed directly into the parenchyma of the brain. Vascular rupture is thought to occur at the small miliary aneurysms, described by Charcot and Bouchard in 1868, and/or at the lipohyalinotic arteries seen frequently in hypertensive patients at autopsy. However, in a minority of cases ICH may be caused by an aneurysm, arteriovenous malformation, cavernous malformation, cerebral amyloid, or a tumor. Glioblastoma is the most frequent primary brain tumor to bleed and melanoma, choriocarcinoma, and hypernephroma are the metastatic tumors that bleed most frequently.

5. The overall mortality from ICH is about 50% with 3/4 of the survivors left with significant neurological deficits. Numerous clinical studies have shown that the prognosis following an ICH depends most on the clinical grade of the patient on admission, its location, and the size of the hemorrhage. Alert patients do much better than comatose patients. In fact a retrospective study by Dixon (1984) demonstrated that the single best predictor of outcome was the Glasgow Coma Scale. Patients with a superficial lobar hemorrhage tend to do better than those with a deeper brain stem hemorrhage. Extension of blood into the ventricular system also worsens the outcome. In addition, patients with a hemorrhage whose measured diameter is greater than 3 cm or whose volume is greater than 50 cc have been shown to do poorly. Patients in poor medical condition and who are greater than 70 years old also tend to have a poor outcome.

The immediate treatment of a patient with an ICH is directed at the control of intracranial pressure and the prevention of further neurological deterioration. Medical measures such as hyperventilation, osmotic diuretics, and steroids are employed to reduce the intracranial hypertension caused by the mass effect of the bleed. The efficacy of surgical intervention is controversial.   There is evidence that the evacuation of large and deeply located hemorrages can increase the survival of comatose patients, especially if done soon after the onset of the bleed.

However these patients are often left with significant neurological deficits.   The patient under discussion showed signs of impending uncal herniation and therefore underwent urgent evacuation of her ICH.   An angiogram, if feasible, allows one to plan for the possibility of encountering a vascular abnormality.   Although the patient made a good recovery and regained consciousness, she was left with a nearly total left hemiplegia.   It therefore seems prudent to seriously <u>consider surgical removal of a large ICH</u>, especially if on the nondominant side, when it is associated   with   persistent   intracranial hypertension   and   continued   neurological deterioration despite maximal medical treatment.

PEARLS:

1. An experimental clinical study by Herbstein and Schaumberg (1974), employing the injection of radioactively   labeled   erythrocytes,   has demonstrated that <u>the active phase of bleeding during an acute ICH lasts for under 2 hours</u>. Subsequent deterioration is therefore thought to be due to reactive brain edema which may be reduced by surgical evacuation of the blood clot.

2. The most frequent artery to bleed is one of the lateral lenticulostriate branches of the middle cerebral artery supplying the putamen.

3. There is currently <u>no evidence that surgery improves the outcome in cases of small ICH</u> without significant mass effect, especially when located superficially in the subcortical white matter.

PITFALLS:

1. When contemplating surgical evacuation of a suspected hypertensive ICH, an <u>angiogram is useful in eliminating other potential causes such as</u>

aneurysm, arteriovenous malformation, or tumor. Unfortunately the possibility of amyloid cannot be reliably predicted and when present may cause intraoperative difficulty in achieving hemostasis. It is also extremely important to test for evidence of a bleeding disorder preoperatively and correct it whenever possible.

2. Cerebellar hemorrhage usually presents without loss of consciousness or motor or sensory deficits. However, headache, dizziness, difficulty walking, and abnormal eye movements frequently occur. Because clinical deterioration can occur rapidly and surgical evacuation has been shown to help some patients, it is important to recognize this clinical entity early.

REFERENCES

1. Ducker TB: Spontaneous intracerebral hemorrhage In Wilkins RH, Rengachary SS, eds. Neurosurgery. New York, McGraw-Hill, 1985, pp 1510-1517.

2. Kase CS, Mohr JP: General features of intracerebral hemorrhage. In Barnett HJM, Mohr JP, Stein BM, Yatsu FM, eds. Stroke, New York, Churchill 1986, pp 497-523.

3. McKissock W, Richardson A, Taylor J: Primary intracerebral hemorrhage: a controlled trial of surgical and conservative treatment in 180 unselected cases. Lancet 2:221-226, 1961.

4. Ropper AH, King AB: Intracranial pressure monitoring in comatose patients with cerebral hemorrhage. Arch Neurol 41:725-728, 1984.

5. Steiner I, Gomori JM, Melamed E: The prognostic value of the CT scan in conservatively treated patients with intracerebral hematoma. Stroke 15(1): 279-282, 1984.

6. Volpin L, Cervellini P, Colombo F, et al: Spontaneous intracerebral hematomas: a new proposal about the usefulness and limits of surgical treatment. Neurosurgery 15(5):663-666, 1984.

OBSTRUCTIVE HYDROCEPHALUS CAUSED BY A MULTI-CYSTIC PARASELLAR MASS

<u>CASE 33</u>: A 45-year-old male presented with a 4 month history of weight loss, headache with occasional diplopia, intermittent nausea and vomiting, and difficulty walking.

The patient was born in Haiti and moved to the United States 5 years ago. He was healthy, having never been hospitalized until 4 months prior to admission. First he noted the onset of a generalized headache which has progressively increased in severity. More recently he has noted increasing nausea and vomiting. Over this period he has had a reduced appetite with a 40 pound weight loss. He has no history of unusual infections or a seizure disorder.

On admission his general physical examination was notable only for the patient being slightly underweight. His neurological examination revealed a slightly blunted affect but otherwise normal mental status with intact memory. Examination of his cranial nerves revealed mild bilateral papilledema with normal visual acuity and grossly normal visual fields. His extraocular movements were full. His sensory examination, motor strength, and reflexes were normal. Testing of his coordination revealed that although his gait was grossly normal, he had difficulty in performing a tandem walk. A Romberg sign was absent.

Computed tomography (CT) and magnetic resonance imaging (MRI) studies revealed marked dilatation of both lateral ventricles with near obliteration of the third ventricle by a multicystic mass filling the parasellar cisterns and compressing the hypothalamus. On CT the mass did not enhance with contrast and calcification was not present.

CLUE: Knowledge of the patient's background (i.e. he grew up in Haiti) and anatomical features of the intracranial mass (see MRI scan) allow the clinician to make an intelligent guess as to the diagnosis.

Figure 33.1

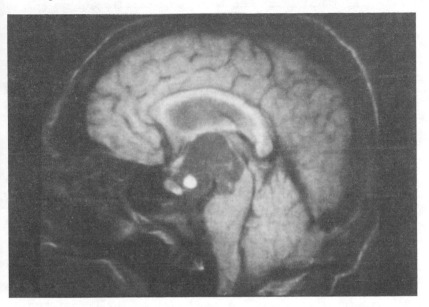

QUESTIONS:

1. What is the differential for masses in this location?

2. What infectious disease common in the tropics could give rise to such a mass?

3. What other studies might be useful?

4. What is the treatment, both surgical and medical, for this condition?

ANSWERS:

1. In order of decreasing frequency, the following masses are found in and around the sella region: <u>pituitary adenoma, meningioma, craniopharyngioma, epidermoid cyst, glioma, metastasis, and parasitic infection</u>. The absence of calcification and failure of this lesion to contrast enhance virtually eliminate all but epidermoid and parasite as possibilities. It is unusual for a cystic epidermoid to cause obstructive hydrocephalus as is evident here. In addition, the mass does have the characteristic appearance of a parasitic infection that, although uncommon in the United States, is prevalent in the tropics as well as South America and parts of the Far East.

2. <u>Cysticercosis, usually from the pork tapeworm Taenia solium, is the most frequent parasite to invade the central nervous system (CNS)</u> in both the tropics and South America. The adult tapeworm resides within the large bowel. However ingested ova, from undercooked pork or contaminated food, can penetrate the mucosa of the small bowel and enter the bloodstream where they may spread to any organ or tissue. The subcutaneous and muscular tissues are most frequently involved followed by the eye and the CNS. In these tissues the ova evolve into an intermediate larval stage, known as the cysticercus, consisting of a cystic bladder portion attached to the scolex, a structure containing several suckers and numerous hook-like appendages. These ova reach the CNS by one of two routes. They can spread via the leptomeningeal vessels to the brain parenchyma and exist as single or multiple lesions. They may also pass via the choroid plexus into the ventricles and on to the cisterns of the brain. It is the location of these lesions that determines their mode of presentation. In this case the patient's signs and symptoms arise from the obstructive hydrocephalus produced by the lesion's near total obliteration of the third ventricle. These parasites can also impede the flow of cerebrospinal fluid (CSF) by inciting a ventriculitis or arachnoiditis depending on their

location.   In addition, intraparenchymal lesions
can cause a local inflammatory response that often
presents as a seizure disorder.

3. It is possible to detect the calcified scolices of
    dead   larvae   on   plain   films   of   the   skull   or
    extremities.   It is important to examine the stool
    of patients suspected of having cysticercosis for
    the presence of adult tapeworms or their ova.   The
    blood   and   CSF   cell   count   can   occasionally
    demonstrate an excess of eosinophils.   Perhaps the
    most specific study is <u>serological testing of the
    blood or CSF</u> for the presence of parasite specific
    antigen.   However, a definite diagnosis can only be
    made   following   excision   of   the   lesion   and   its
    pathological examination under the microscope.

4. The surgical management of this patient is directed
    first at relieving the obstructive hydrocephalus by
    placement of a ventriculoperitoneal shunt.   There
    is   no   evidence   that   shunting   disseminates   the
    disease.   After treating the hydrocephalus surgery
    should then be directed at removing the lesion.   In
    this   case   a   frontotemporal   craniotomy   provides
    sufficient exposure to remove the lesion.   Extreme
    care should be taken to avoid breaking the cysts,
    the spillage of whose contents can incite a severe
    inflammatory response.   The use of intraoperative
    steroids   provides   an   additional   measure   of
    protection.   As an adjunct to surgery <u>the drug
    Praziquantel has been introduced for the treatment
    of disseminated cysticercosis</u>.   It is of particular
    importance in cases where incomplete removal of the
    parasite is suspected.

PEARLS:

1. As in this case, several years may elapse between
    exposure of the patient to the parasite and the
    onset of symptoms.

2. The detection of cysticercosis in the subcutaneous
    tissues   or   muscles   strongly   suggests   CNS
    involvement.

3. The most common extraparenchymal and extraventricular location of cysticercosis is within the basal cisterns in a racemose pattern as exemplified by this case.

PITFALLS:

1. Total excision of the parasitic lesion should always be attempted. Even in cases where the scolex is dead, the cyst wall is capable of continuing to grow unless completely removed.

2. The drug Praziquantel should always be used in conjunction with steroids to reduce the severity of inflammation caused by the death of the larval parasites.

REFERENCES

1. Beaver PC, Jung RC, Cupp EW: Clinical parasitology, Philadelphia, Lea and Febiger, 1984, pp 512-519.

2. Berman JD, Beaver PC, Cheever AW, et al: Cysticercus of 60 millileter volume in human brain. Am J Trop Med Hyg 30(3):616-619, 1981.

3. Priestley SE, Wiles PG: Cysticercosis-induced epilepsy diagnosed by computerized tomography. J Soc Occup Med 29:149-150, 1979.

4. Stern ES: Parasitic infections, in Wilkins, RH and Rengachary SS eds. Neurosurgery, New York, McGraw-Hill, 1985 pp 2010-2015.

5. Jung RC, Rodriguez MA, Beaver PC, et al: Racemose cysticercus in human brain. Am J Trop Med Hyg 30(3):620-624, 1981.

SURGICAL INTERN WITH HEADACHE

<u>CASE 34:</u> A 25-year-old surgical intern in a busy
hospital began to complain of headache. He went to his
chief residents and said that he did not feel well.
They said, "Tough!" His headache became worse over the
next month. He went to his chief residents and said
that his headaches were worse and he could not do his
job. They said, "Still Tough!" Two weeks later he
developed nausea and projectile vomiting. He was
brought to the emergency room where examination was
normal except for bilateral papilledema. A computed
tomography (CT) scan was obtained.

Clue: Figure 34.1   CT scan

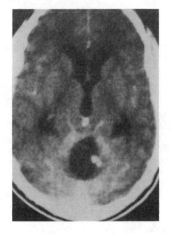

QUESTIONS:

1. What is wrong with this man?

2. Could anything else present this way?

3. Is this an isolated condition?

4. How would you investigate him?

5. What would you do?

6. What is his prognosis?

ANSWERS:

1.   This man has all of the symptoms and signs of a
     <u>posterior fossa mass lesion</u>. The commonest benign
     cystic cerebellar tumors in adults are
     <u>hemangioblastomas</u>. They are benign tumors of blood
     vessels. They present as posterior fossa lesions
     some 70% of which are cystic. They may occur
     elsewhere in the central nervous system;
     specifically supratentorially, where they are
     usually (80%) solid and rare enough to be
     reportable and in the spinal cord, where they make
     up approximately 2% of all neoplasms.

2.   This is the presentation of any posterior fossa
     mass. It could, for instance, be an ependymoma,
     astrocystoma or, rarer in this age group, a
     medulloblastoma or metastasis. This man had a
     cerebellar hemangioblastoma.

3.   Cerebellar hemangioblastomas were described as such
     by Cushing and Bailey who realized that they were
     blood vessel tumors. In 1904 Von Hippel had
     described 2 patients with <u>retinal masses associated
     with dilated retinal vasculature and detachment</u>,
     concluding that these masses were
     hemangioblastomas. When one died, an autopsy
     revealed tumors in the cerebellum, base of the
     brain, and cauda equina. There were renal,
     pancreatic, and epididymal cysts and kidney and
     bladder tumors. In 1926 Arvid Lindau, a Swedish
     pathologist who was investigating cerebellar cysts,
     found that these cysts were often associated with
     pancreatic and renal cysts and with renal cell
     carcinoma. He characterized the pathology of the
     cerebellar cysts, describing the 3 types of cells
     involved, the endothelial, the pericyte, and the
     stromal cell. <u>Von Hippel-Lindau syndrome is an
     autosomal dominant disorder with mixed penetrance
     characterized by hemangioblastomas of the central
     nervous system (frequently multiple), retinal
     hemangioblastomas, renal cell carcinoma (25%),
     pheochromocytoma (10%), and multiple other benign
     and malignant cystic conditions of the viscerae</u>.
     Hemangioblastomas may occur either sporadically or
     as part of this syndrome.

4. CT with contrast is the best screening test,
    although it is not as sensitive as vertebral
    angiography in detecting small posterior fossa
    lesions. This should be done in someone suspected
    of Von Hippel-Lindau.

5. The treatment of this benign condition is surgery.
    The cysts all have a solid nodule which must be
    removed. The solid tumors should be treated as if
    they were vascular malformations and removed in
    toto. The solid elements of these tumors consist
    of a meshwork of anastomosing capillary structures.
    Radiation therapy is not indicated unless the tumor
    is inoperable.

6. The prognosis depends on the position of the tumors
    and the associated Von Hippel-Lindau syndrome.
    Solid tumors and brain stem tumors have higher
    operative mortality while multiple tumors and the
    associated renal carcinoma make the prognosis more
    guarded in Von Hippel-Lindau if it is present.

    This patient had a sporadic cystic cerebellar
    tumor which was resected and he has had no problem
    since. The prognosis in such cases is excellent.

PEARLS:

1. The cerebellar cysts are really pseudocysts, being
    lined with compressed normal tissue. The solid
    mural nodule exudes fluid which forms the cyst.
    Therefore drainage of the cyst alone without
    removal of the mural nodule results in rapid
    reaccumulation.

2. This patient's hematocrit was 60%. Polycythemia is
    thought to be due to the secretion of
    erythropoietin by the tumor, but no one knows.

3. Intratumoral hemorrhages are rare in patients with
    cerebellar hemangioblastomas.

PITFALLS:

1. All patients with cerebellar hemangioblastomas must be evaluated for Von Hippel-Lindau syndrome.

2. The second most common site for hemangioblastomas is the spinal cord and occasionally there may be an associated syrinx.

3. The return or persistence of polycythemia after the surgical resection of a hemangioblastoma indicates an incomplete removal or another untreated lesion.

4. Hemangioblastomas may have a similar angiographic appearance of hemangiopericytomas, angioblastic meningiomas, or arteriovenous malformations.

REFERENCES

1. Rengechary S: In Wilkins R, Rengechary S eds: Neurosurgery. New York, McGraw-Hill, pp 772-782, 1985.

2. Jeffreys R: Clinical and surgical aspects of posterior fossa hemangioblastomas. J Neurol Neurosurg Psych 38:105-111, 1975.

3. Diehl P, Symon L: Supratentorial intraventricular hemangioblastoma. Case report and review of the literature. Surg Neurol 15:435-443, 1981.

PULSATING EYE AND DECREASED VISION AFTER AN ACCIDENT

CASE 35: A 34-year-old man struck his head on a
windshield during a motor vehicle collision. The
patient did not lose consciousness or sustain any other
injuries at the time and was released from an emergency
room after a suitable period of observation. Shortly
thereafter he noted a steady pulsation of his left eye
which was associated with a throbbing sound within his
head. He sought medical evaluation when he noted a
steady progression in these symptoms in addition to
reddening of his left eye, mildly decreased vision of
the eye, and double vision when looking to his left
side.

Neuroanatomical Clue:

Figure 35.1:

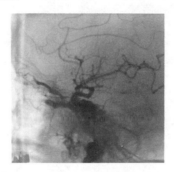

The cavernous sinus, which contains the carotid
artery, is in direct communication with several venous
plexuses, both intra- and extracranially.

QUESTIONS:

1. What is the diagnosis?

2. How do you account for this patient's symptoms and
signs?

3. Is this a life threatening condition?

4. How would you confirm the diagnosis?

5. What treatments can be offered to this patient?

ANSWERS:

1.   <u>The patient has a carotid cavernous fistula</u>.   A
     carotid cavernous fistula (CCF) is created by a
     direct communication between the intracavernous
     sinus portion of the carotid artery and the venous
     plexus which surrounds it.   There are many
     mechanisms by which such a communication can form
     with the most common being posttraumatic as in
     this case.   <u>Other etiologies include direct</u>
     <u>penetration of the carotid artery and venous plexus</u>
     <u>in the cavernous sinus by a foreign object or</u>
     <u>during a surgical procedure, rupture of a carotid</u>
     <u>artery aneurysm within the sinus, or spontaneous</u>
     <u>creation of fistula without proceeding trauma or</u>
     <u>obvious pathology</u>.

     The diagnosis is usually established proceeding
     a traumatic event after which the patient notices a
     pulsation of one or both eyes, an audible bruit in
     the head, protrusion and reddening of the eye,
     decreased vision, double vision, and headache.

2.   The symptoms and physical signs of a CCF are
     produced by the anatomy of the cavernous sinus.
     Although controversy exists concerning the precise
     anatomical relationships between arteries and veins
     within the sinus, the principle concept is that the
     carotid artery before it enters the subarachnoid
     space of the brain is enclosed in a dural cavity on
     either side of the sella turcica that contains a
     network of veins and the following cranial nerves:
     III, IV, VI, V1, and V2.   <u>The veins of the</u>
     <u>cavernous sinus are in direct communication with</u>
     <u>the veins of the opposite cavernous sinus, superior</u>
     <u>ophthalmic vein, and the posterior fossa basilar</u>
     <u>venous plexus through numerous anastomotic venous</u>
     <u>channels within the dura of the skull base</u>.   A
     situation which creates a direct carotid to venous
     plexus communication within the cavernous sinus
     (fistula) will contain the blood flow from the
     carotid and shunt this flow usually to the superior
     ophthalmic vein.   This <u>increased blood flow and</u>
     <u>pressure from the fistula in the cavernous sinus to</u>
     <u>the orbit via the superior ophthalmic vein creates</u>
     <u>the observed symptoms</u>.   This leads directly to

pulsations in the orbit, a bruit, exophthalmos, or
injury to the cranial nerves in the cavernous
sinus.   Decreased vision is usually created by
retinal artery ischemia secondary to increased
retinal venous pressure from the fistula.

3.   Despite the high blood flows seen in a CCF the
condition is rarely life threatening as the fistula
is contained completely within the walls of the
cavernous sinus and thus separate from the brain
and its subarachnoid space.

4.   The procedure of choice both for diagnosis and
therapy is an angiogram.   The angiogram will
document the presence and size of a fistula, the
channels of venous drainage, possible etiology of
the fistula, and the best method of therapy.

5.   CCF may be treated by intravascular embolization
techniques or by direct surgical attack.
Embolization is usually accomplished at the same
time as the diagnostic angiogram and involves
placing a small balloon within the carotid artery
at the point of its connection with the venous
plexus within the cavernous sinus.   This is a
highly effective and safe technique when done by
experienced neuroradiologists and can be used in
the majority of CCF.   Occasionally direct surgical
obliteration of the fistula or its venous outflow
is required but these are complex approaches that
should be reserved when embolization techniques are
not successful.   Rarely will a CCF
spontaneously resolve, sometimes after the
diagnostic angiogram, particularly if the fistula
is small.

PEARLS:

1.   The VIth cranial nerve, because of its location
within the cavernous sinus, is twice as often
affected as the cranial nerves contained within the
walls of the cavernous sinus (III, IV, V1, and V2).

2.   Spontaneous CCFs are less common than posttraumatic
     CCFs. Spontaneous CCFs usually occur in middle-
     aged or postmenopausal women. These tend to be
     unilateral and are thought to be due to
     arteriovenous malformations within the dural leaves
     of the cavernous sinus. Although the flow and
     pressure of these fistulas is less than
     posttraumatic CCFs, they can be difficult to treat
     as several small fistulas may be created and blood
     supply may be from both the internal and external
     carotid arteries.

3.   A rare cause of a CCF is rupture of a wholly
     intracavernous carotid artery aneurysm.

4.   The spontaneous remission rate of CCF is estimated
     to be 5-10% of cases.

PITFALLS:

1.   The differential diagnosis of a protruding,
     pulsatile eye should always include a congenital
     absence of the sphenoid wing as seen in
     neurofibromatosis. In this condition the dura of
     the temporal lobe is in contact with the orbital
     tissues because of a defect in the sphenoid bone
     and the brain pulsations can be transmitted to the
     orbit directly, resulting in a pulsatile
     exopthalmus.

2.   Other conditions that may have the symptoms of a
     CCF include: cavernous sinus thrombosis, endocrine
     (thyroid) exophthalmos, retro-orbital tumors, or
     orbital vascular malformations.

3.   In a small percentage of cases, the CCF will drain
     to the posterior fossa venous plexus and the eyes
     may not be involved.

4.   Because both cavernous sinuses are in communication
     with one another through anastomotic veins coursing
     around the sella turcia, a CCF in one eye may shunt
     blood to the opposite cavernous sinus thereby
     producing similar symptoms on the uninvolved side.
     These patients will present with bilateral
     pulsatile exopthalmus.

REFERENCES

1. Barrow DL, Spector RH, Braun IF, et al:
   Classification and treatment of spontaneous carotid
   cavernous sinus fistulas. J Neurosurg 62:248-
   256, 1985.

2. Debrun G, LaCour P, Carar J, et al: Detachable
   balloon and calibrated balloon techniques in the
   treatments of cerebrovascular lesions. J
   Neurosurg 49:635-649, 1978.

3. Hamby WB: Carotid cavernous fistulas. Springfield,
   IL, Charles C Thomas, 1966.

4. Isamat F, Ferrer E, Tnose J: Direct intracavernous
   obliteration of high flow carotid cavernous
   fistulas. J Neurosurg 65:770-775, 1986.

5. Newton TH, and Hoyt WF: Dural arteriovenous shunts
   in the region of the cavernous sinus. Neuroradiology
   1:71-81, 1970.

6. Parkinson D: A surgical approach to the cavernous
   portion of the carotid artery: anatomical studies
   and case report. J Neurosurg 23:474-483, 1965.

HYPERTENSIVE MAN WITH TRANSIENT NEUROLOGICAL DYSFUNCTION

CASE 36: A 67-year-old man presented to his physician after having experienced 1-2 minutes of transient right hand numbness and incoordination associated with word-finding difficulty the previous day. The patient had a history of hypertension diagnosed 12 years previously and was currently being treated with a diuretic and propranolol. He had recently quit smoking after 40 years of 1-2 packs per day of cigarette smoking. Approximately 2 months prior to presentation the patient experienced similar symptoms but did not seek medical attention.

On examination the patient appeared well. The blood pressure was 150/90 and the heart rate 60 beats per minute. The fundi showed some arteriolar narrowing but were otherwise unremarkable. Examination of the neck revealed no bruits. The heart, lungs, abdomen, and extremities were unremarkable. Neurological examination revealed no abnormalities.

QUESTIONS:

1. At this point what is your differential diagnosis and what diagnostic test or tests would you order next?

2. A computed tomography scan of the head with and without intravenous contrast was normal. Echocardiography showed only mild left ventricular hypertrophy. Doppler studies of the carotid arteries showed an approximately 90% stenosis on the left. Cerebral angiography demonstrated a high grade stenosis at the bifurcation of the left common carotid artery (see Fig. 36.1).

206

Figure 36.1: Left common carotid angiogram.

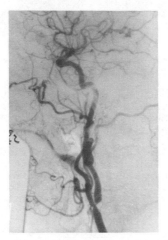

Note the high grade stenosis of the internal carotid artery at the bifurcation of the common carotid artery.

What is your diagnosis now? Describe the pathophysiology believed to account for this disease state.

3. What treatment modalities are available for this patient? Consider the advantages and disadvantages of each form of treatment.

4. Discuss the significance of cervical bruits on the management of atherosclerotic cerebrovascular disease.

ANSWERS:

1.   The differential diagnosis in this patient is not extensive. The most obvious diagnosis is, of course, <u>transient cerebral ischemia in the distribution of the left middle cerebral artery</u>. It is important, however, to first obtain a computed tomography (CT) scan of the head with and without intravenous contrast to rule out a mass lesion. Mass lesions such as primary or metastatic tumors, abscesses, vascular anomalies, or even intracranial hemorrhages may present initially with transient focal symptoms.

   In the evaluation of patients with suspected transient cerebral ischemia, attention must be directed to the evaluation of their cardiac and cerebrovascular systems. Echocardiography is used to detect possible cardiac embolic sources. Doppler ultrasonography is a noninvasive method of evaluating the patency of the carotid arteries but <u>angiography continues to be the definitive imaging technique</u> for evaluation of the carotid arteries.

2.   This patient suffered from transient neurological dysfunction referable to the left cerebral hemisphere in the vascular distribution of the middle cerebral artery. Episodes such as these are typical of <u>transient ischemic attacks (TIAs)</u>. TIAs are episodes of focal neurological deficit caused by cerebral ischemia and lasting less than 24 hours. They represent one end of a spectrum of cerebral ischemia at the other end of which is cerebral infarction and completed stroke. <u>Reversible ischemia neurological deficits (RINDs)</u> are focal neurological symptoms or signs which last 24 to 48 hours.

   TIAs may be manifested by a variety of neurological symptoms. If the ischemia is in the vascular distribution of the carotid arteries (i.e., the anterior cerebral circulation; including the ophthalmic artery, the anterior cerebral artery, and the middle cerebral artery) the symptoms may include <u>transient monocular blindness (amaurosis fugax)</u>, weakness or sensory changes in an extremity or on one side of the body or face, disturbances of language or cognition, and other symptoms. Symptoms such as vertigo, nausea, ataxia, dysarthria, diplopia, and dysphagia when transient may represent ischemia in the territory of the vertebral-basilar circulation (i.e., the posterior circulation). Symptoms of lightheadedness or "dizziness" without vertigo, although possibly indicative of generalized cerebral ischemia, are not suffiently localizing to be considered symptomatic of TIAs.

The etiology of TIAs is not entirely clear. It was once thought that carotid artery stenosis resulting in insufficient or variable cerebral blood flow caused the symptomatology and indeed it may in some cases. Current theory, however, considers artery to artery emboli to be the cause of the majority of TIAs. These emboli may arise from any source between the heart and brain and may include emboli from atrial myxomas or mitral valve vegetations in subacute bacterial endocarditis or rarely peripheral venous emboli in patients with atrial or ventricular septal defects. More frequently the origin of the emboli is thought to be from atheromatous plaques occurring at or near the bifurcation of the common carotid arteries. Platelet-fibrin aggregates and/or cholesterol fragments may embolize to the brain especially from those plaques which appear ulcerated on angiography. These emboli lodge in the small arterioles of the brain or retina obstructing blood flow and thus causing localizing symptoms. The symptoms are transient because the emboli may break up and disperse or small collateral vascular channels may open as a result of the focal ischemia and provide sufficient blood flow to alleviate the symptoms. In the case of transient monocular blindness cholesterol emboli have actually been visualized in the retinal circulation.

TIA's can be treated by medical or surgical means. Despite substantial literature on the subject there is, as yet, no definite treatment of choice as determined by randomized, prospective, clinical trials. <u>Medical therapy consists of anticoagulation and antiplatelet therapy</u>. Anticoagulation therapy is effective in treating emboli of cardiac origin and possibly in decreasing the frequency of vertebral-basilar TIAs.

Drugs that interfere with the adhesiveness of platelets have recently emerged in the treatment of TIAs and the prevention of stroke. <u>That platelet inhibition is effective in preventing TIA and stroke lends support to the platelet-fibrin thromboembolic theory of TIA</u>. Several major randomized, prospective studies have demonstrated the efficacy of aspirin in the treatment of TIAs and the prevention of stroke. Aspirin appears to interfere with platelet aggregation by inhibiting prostaglandin synthesis. Other antiplatelet aggregation medications work by inhibiting prostaglandin synthesis. Other antiplatelet agents such as dipyridamole and sulfinpyrazone have not been shown to be effective in TIA or stroke prevention. Initially the protective effect of aspirin was thought to be limited to men but subsequent studies have demonstrated a benefit in women as well. It appears that the reduction in stroke achieved with aspirin is from 30 to 50%. The aforementioned studies used large doses of aspirin (1000-1300 mg/day). There is a theoretical advantage to using smaller doses of aspirin for the prevention of TIA and stroke. It is proposed that smaller doses of aspirin may spare the inhibition of antiaggregatory prostacycline while still inhibiting proaggregatory thromboxane A_2. Trials are currently underway to determine the clinical usefulness of this idea.

<u>Surgical therapy for TIAs of the anterior circulation consists primarily of carotid endarterectomy</u>. Other cerebrorevascularization procedures such as extracranial to intracranial bypass are reserved for special circumstances. During carotid endarterectomy the atheromatous plaque is removed directly via carotid arteriotomy.

The technique can be performed under general or local anesthesia. When done under general anesthesia electroencephalographic (EEG) monitoring can be helpful in detecting intraoperative cerebral ischemia. Often a shunt is used to continue cerebral blood flow on the operated side during the procedure. Indications for the use of a shunt are controversial. Some surgeons use a shunt routinely whereas others rarely do. Should collateral cerebral blood flow be compromised, however, most surgeons consider the use of a shunt.

Carotid endarterectomy has been shown in prospective studies performed in the late 1960s and early 1970s to decrease TIA symptoms and the rate of subsequent stroke. However, the surgical morbidity and mortality of these studies was high at 11-24%. Operative morbidity has since improved and currently major centers report morbidity and mortality of <3%.

4. Cervical bruits occur in approximately 4% of the population 40 years of age or older. The prevalence increases with age and the presence of hypertension. Although cervical bruits usually indicate the presence of carotid stenosis, this stenosis is not always significant. In patients with cervical bruits and no TIA or stroke symptoms the overall stroke rate is 2%. In these patients, however, subsequent stroke location correlates poorly with the side of the bruit. A subgroup of patients with cervical bruits and severely stenotic carotid arteries are at an increased risk of stroke.

   Persons with asymptomatic carotid bruits have a myocardial ischemic rate of 7% per year and an annual mortality of 4%, mostly from heart disease. As such, the presence of carotid artery bruits in a patient without neurological symptoms should be regarded as a marker for generalized atherosclerotic vascular disease and not considered an indication for carotid surgery. Patients with carotid bruits should, however, have ultrasonic or angiographic evaluation to determine the degree of stenosis present.

PEARLS:

There have been many epidemiological studies regarding cervical bruits and TIAs and the risks of stroke, myocardial infarction, and death. The literature is profuse and confusing. The following comments represent a distillation of results of the major studies.

1. Both TIAs and cervical bruits are predictors of generalized atherosclerotic disease. In patients with TIAs, cardiac ischemic disease is more than twice as likely as stroke to be the cause of death.

2. In patients with asymptomatic bruits the annual stroke rate is 2%, the myocardial ischemic rate is 7%, and the annual mortality is 4%. The correlation between that side of the bruit and the side of subsequent stroke is poor.

3. In patients with TIAs, the annual stroke rate is 5 to 10% and the annual mortality is 6%.

REFERENCES

1. Patterson RH: Can carotid endarterectomy be justified? Yes. Arch Neurol 44:651-2, 1987.

2. Chambers BR, Norris JW: Outcome of patients with asymptomatic neck bruits. N Engl J Med 315:860-865, 1986.

3. Fields WS: Aspirin for prevention of stroke: a review. Am J Med 74(6A):61-65, 1983.

4. Crowell RM, Ojemann RG: Surgical management of extracranial occlusive disease in stroke: pathophysiology, diagnosis and management. eds. Barnett HJM, Mohr JP, Stein BM, Yatsu FM, New York, Churchill Livingston, 1986 p 1003.

CHILD WITH STAGGERING GAIT

CASE 37: This 6-year-old boy developed progressive ·
difficulty walking over the last 4 weeks. His parents
noted that he had a staggering gait and had grown
clumsy with his right hand. He complained of headaches
for the last 3 months and for the last week awakened
every day with nausea and vomiting which improved later
in the day.

On examination he had bilateral papilledema and
bilateral VIth nerve palsies. He also had nystagmus on
lateral gaze. His gait was markedly ataxic and wide-
based, and he had dysmetria with his right hand. Plain
skull film showed separation of the sutures. The
computed tomography (CT) scan showed a midline
hyperdense contrast enhancing cerebellar tumor. There
was dramatic ventricular dilation with periventricular
edema (see Fig. 37.1 - contrast CT scan).

Clue:

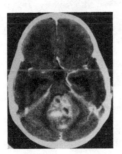

Figure 37.1

QUESTIONS:

1. Give a differential diagnosis for this tumor.
   Correlate this with radiological findings.

2. Correlate the clinical features seen in this child
   with the tumor's location.

3. Describe the gross and microscopic pathology of
   medulloblastomas.

4. Describe treatment modalities and outcome for
   medulloblastomas.

ANSWERS:

1.   The most likely diagnosis based on the history,
     neurological examination, and radiographic findings
     is medulloblastoma. Medulloblastomas account to 15
     to 20 percent of central nervous system (CNS)
     tumors in children; 70 % occur in patients
     less than 8 years of age but they have been
     reported up to the seventh decade. On noncontrast
     CT scan they appeared variegated, isodense to
     hyperdense, and tended to fill the IVth ventricle.
     They contain calcium and cysts less often than
     other posterior fossa tumors, and are uniformly
     enhancing. Posterior fossa astrocytomas constitute
     10 to 20 percent of childhood brain tumors. They
     are more commonly located in the cerebellar
     hemisphere than the vermis, tonsils, or brain stem.
     They characteristically have a lower density than
     brain, commonly have cysts, and enhance with
     contrast. Twenty-two percent will have associated
     calcifications.

        Ependymomas account for approximately 10% of
     pediatric posterior fossa tumors. They are
     isodense or slightly hyperdense with thin well
     defined, low attenuation halo around the tumor.
     Contrast enhancement is inhomogeneous. Cysts are
     common. Obstructive hydrocephalus is present in 90%
     of patients. Calcifications are seen in over 50%
     of ependymomas (versus 10% of medulloblastomas).

        Choroid plexus papillomas are more common in the
     lateral ventricles in children. There is marked
     hydrocephalus and marked contrast enhancement.

        In addition to the above, posterior fossa tumors
     may include hemangioblastomas, metastatic disease,
     cerebellar abscesses, arachnoid cysts, epidermoids,
     and subependymal astrocytomas.

2.   The IVth ventricle is the preferred site for
     medulloblastomas and they most commonly present
     with signs of increased intracranial pressure
     secondary to obstruction of flow of ceberospinal
     fluid (CSF). Morning headaches, nausea, and
     vomiting are common. As the child sleeps, there is

a decrease in venous drainage and an increase in $PaCO_2$ which results in increased intracranial pressure. As the child rises venous drainage improves; with vomiting, there is hyperventilation and a decrease in $PaCO_2$.

There is associated bilateral papilledema and often bilateral VIth nerve palsies as a result of the marked hydrocephalus and increased intracranial pressure. Because of vermian involvement, there are midline cerebellar symptoms. With asymmetric extension, there may also be unilateral cerebellar findings.

3.   Medulloblastomas are usually located midline in the posterior fossa and adherent to the posterior medullar velum of the IVth ventricle. They are reddish, priable, and often quite vascular in appearance. Fifteen percent show evidence of recent or old hemorrhage at the time of surgery. They are embryonal tumors, originating from primitive poorly differentiated cells that arise immediately above the IVth ventricle, and migrate over the cerebellum during gestation. They may be intimately adherent to the anterior medullar velum, the aquaduct, or the floor of the IVth ventricle.

A distinct subtype of medulloblastomas are desmoplastic medulloblastomas. They are found in older patients (greater than 20 years of age) and are located laterally in the cerebellar hemisphere. Particularly in the older patient, these tumors have a better prognosis.

4.   Initial management consists of diversion of CSF and relief of hydrocephalus, either with placement of a ventriculoperitoneal shunt or a ventricular drain. An important feature of medulloblastoma is their tendency to spread via the CSF pathways. There have been reports of peritoneal seeding by medulloblastomas via ventriculoperitoneal shunts. Some investigators have advocated placement of filter devices but these result in a significant rate of shunt malfunction. Another concern with shunting is that if there is a sudden decrease in pressure in the supratentorial compartment, there

may be upward herniation by the posterior fossa tumor. Some investigators report up to a 4% incidence of upward herniation and advocate the more gradual decrease in pressure afforded by a ventricular drain or treatment with high dose corticosteroids to decrease intracranial pressure.

Surgery is performed via a posterior fossa craniectomy. Particular attention is paid to infiltration of the tumor into the floor of the IVth ventricle. Following surgery radiation therapy is given: 4000 to 4500 rads to the whole cranial cavity and 3000 to 4000 to the spinal axis. Whole neuroaxia radiation is given because of the high propensity of CSF spread by the tumor. Because of the devastating effects of radiation therapy to the developing brain, young children are not given radiation therapy but receive chemotherapy instead. Recent studies suggest a beneficial effect of chemotherapy, but long term results have not been encouraging.

The 5-year survival for this tumor varies between 25 and 70% and is correlated with total surgical excision followed by radiation therapy. In younger patients (less than 2 years) 100% mortality can be expected. In assessing the period of risk Collin's law is employed. The period of risk encompasses a time equal to the patients age at diagnosis plus 9 months.

PEARLS:

1. Medulloblastomas account to 15 to 20% of brain tumors in children and are most common in the first decade of life.

2. Medulloblastomas classically produce signs of increased intracranial pressure secondary to hydrocephalus and midline cerebellar symptoms secondary to vermian involvement.

3. Diversion of CSF by shunt or ventricular drain provides important relief of life-threatening hydrocephalus.

4. Five year survival rates, as reported by major
    pediatric neurosurgical institutions, after surgery
    and radiotherapy are between 40 and 60%.

PITFALLS:

1. Medulloblastomas can metastasize via CSF pathways
    throughout the central nervous system. They
    produce a characteristic "sugar coating" because of
    tumor spread in the subarachnoid space.

2. Up to a 19% extracranial metastasis rate is
    reported after shunting.

3. Rapid decompression of the posterior fossa can
    result in upward herniation necessitating emergent
    posterior fossa decompression and removal of the
    tumor.

4. Brain stem infiltration occurs in up to 30-40% of
    patients.

5. There is a high incidence (80-90%) of low
    intelligence quotient (IQ) scores and behavioral
    disorder in children treated with medulloblastoma.
    There is also an associated high incidence of
    growth retardation (60%). These complications are
    related to radiation therapy and surgery and the
    tumor's effects on the developing brain.

REFERENCES

1. Berry MP, Jenkin RDT, Keen DW, et al: Radiation
   treatment for medulloblastoma.   A 21 year review. J
   Neurosurg 55:43-51, 1981.

2. Hirsch JF, Renier C, Czernichow P, et al:
   Medulloblastoma in childhood.   Survival and
   functional results.   Acta Neurochir 48:1-15, 1979.

3. Park TS, Hoffman HJ, Hendrick EB, et al:
   Medulloblastoma: clinical presentation and
   management. J Neurosurg 58:543-552, 1983.

4. Quest DO, Brisman R, Antunes JL, et al: Period of
   risk for recurrence in medulloblastoma. J Neurosurg
   48:159-163, 1978.

5. Raimondi AJ, Tomita T: Medulloblastoma in childhood:
   comparative results of partial and total resection.
   Childs Brain 5:310-328, 1979.

6. Schut L, Bruce DA, Sutton LN: Medulloblastomas. In
   Wilkins RH, Rengachary SS, eds: Neurosurgery.
   New York, McGraw-Hill, 1985, pp 758-762.

MAN WITH LOW BACK PAIN

CASE 38: A 60-year-old diabetic man presents with a 3-week history of midback pain. He had come to the emergency room on three separate occasions complaining of back pain and was given a diagnosis of paraspinal muscle spasm. Plain x-rays repeated at each visit were negative. His neurological exam was normal. Chemistry and complete blood count (CBC) were entirely within normal limits. He was treated with muscle relaxants and analgesics.

On the date of admission he awakened with severe back and paraspinal muscle pain in the upper lumbar region. He noted that his legs were weak and that he could no longer walk. He had a fever ($101.6^{\circ}F$). Neurological examination was remarkable for decreased strength in both lower extremities, increased lower extremity reflexes, with bilateral Babinski reflexes. There was decreased sensation to all modalities from T_{10} down. General physical examination was remarkable for a recently healed foot ulcer. He had point tenderness on palpation of his spine at the T_{12} to L_2 region and nuchal pain with cervical extension and flexion.

Complete spine films were consistent with degenerative joint disease without evidence of metastatic disease or bony erosion. A myelogram was performed with metrizamide and was followed by a computed tomography (CT) scan. A complete block secondary to epidural compression was seen from T_{10} to L_2. CT scan suggested a paraspinal mass at T_{11} to L_1. Blood work revealed an elevated white blood cell count (WBC) of 12 (per cubic millimeter), and an erythrocyte sedimentation rate (ESR) of 80. The cerebrospinal fluid (CSF) profile revealed a white count of 300, protein of 120, and glucose of 55.

CLUE:

The epidural space is diagrammed below and contains a rich venous plexus. Note that the blood supply to the cord is supplied by one anterior spinal artery and two posterior spinal arteries.

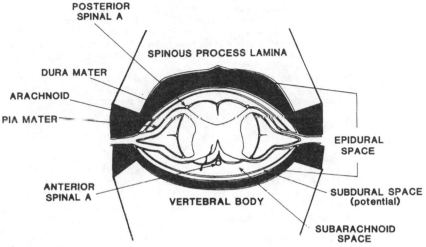

Figure 38.1

QUESTIONS:

1. What is the differential diagnosis in this case?
   Describe some of the findings for each of the
   diagnoses suggested.

2. What are the laboratory findings in such patients?

3. What radiographic tests might be appropriate and
   what would they offer in the way of information?

4. What organisms are commonly seen? What are the
   possible origins of this infection?

5. Describe treatment modalities for spinal epidural
   abscess and possible outcome?

ANSWERS:

1. This patient presents with a history of several weeks of back pain followed by the sudden development of neurological deficits. The radiological studies suggest epidural compression of the cauda equina. Among the diseases which must be considered initially is <u>metastatic tumor with primarily epidural extension</u>. Signs of systemic disease are usually present with metastatic disease with bony changes frequently evident on plain spine films. Osteomyelitis usually presents with back pain and may, with vertebral collapse, have signs of spinal cord compression. There are, however, usually plain film changes suggestive of bony erosion. Acute transverse myelitis may also present with a sudden paralysis over 72 hours. Pain is usually absent (less than 37% have pain) and the myelogram is normal or shows mild cord edema. <u>Intramedullary spinal cord tumors have a progressive course and show radiographic evidence of cord enlargement</u>.

    Spinal epidural abscess must be considered in patients who are immunosuppressed, intravenous (IV) drug abusers, diabetics, or have systemic infection, and who present with persistent back pain without a clear etiology. <u>The pain is usually localized with point tenderness and fever may be present</u>. Their neurological deficits are referable to the level of the lesion.

2. Patients with epidural abscess are divided into two groups: those with acute presentation (symptoms less than 2 weeks) and those with a more chronic presentation (greater than 2 weeks of symptoms). Those patients with acute presentations most consistently show an elevated white blood cell count.

    In those with a more chronic process, such as that seen in this patient, the white blood cell count may be normal or slightly elevated.

    <u>Cerebrospinal fluid shows a parameningeal infectious process</u>. WBC count is slightly elevated (mean of 60 per cubic millimeter) with

polymorphonuclear leukocytes and lymphocytes in equal proportions. There is an elevated protein particularly below the level of the block and the glucose is often normal.

ESR is consistently elevated in both the acute and chronic groups.

3. Radiographic tests begin with a set of plain spine films which are normal in 50-75% of the cases.

The myelogram is the most sensitive radiographic examination and reveals abnormalities in greater than 95% of patients. There is a picture of an epidural mass with partial or complete block to the flow of contrast medium. The myelogram frequently reveals multiple levels of involvement.

Computed tomography (CT) scans in addition to demonstrating epidural compression may reveal a contiguous paraspinal abscess collection such as in the psoas muscle.

Bone scans may help reveal uptake with adjacent vertebral bodies suggesting osteomyelitis despite negative plain films. It is unusual for bone scans to be negative in the face of an epidural abscess.

Magnetic resonance imaging (MRI) scan has only recently been used and it reveals an epidural collection with evidence of cord edema.

4. Staphylococcus aureus is found in over 50% of the epidural infections and greater than 75% of the infections are caused by gram-positive aerobic cocci. Next in order of frequency are aerobic Streptococci, Staphylococcus epidermidis, Escherisia coli, Enterobacter aerogenes, Pseudomonas, and Haemophilus. More than one organism can be seen. Blood cultures are positive in 50-60% of the patients.

Recent studies suggest that in 20-30% of the patients no clear source of infection could be identified. Associated sources of infection included skin or soft tissue infection (such as diabetic foot ulcers), recent spinal surgery or procedures, pulmonary infections, urinary tract infections, IV drug abuse, and recent trauma.

5. Treatment is based upon identification of the organism and treatment with appropriate antibiotics. When neurological deficits occur, particularly spinal cord compression, decompressive laminectomy may be indicated.

At surgery purulent material is usually seen only in patients with an acute presentation. In more chronic cases, granulation tissue is often found at surgery with evidence of epidural scarring. In 5-10% of patients no organism is found and in those patients presumptive antibiotic coverage must include anti-staphylococcal treatment. Gram negative organisms must be considered with a history of recent spinal procedure or IV drug abuse.

Outcome is clearly related to age of the patient, presenting medical condition and neurological status. Improvement following surgical intervention is dependent on the duration of neurological deficit prior to surgery.

The cause of neurological deficit has been speculated to be either secondary to inflammation of the epidural space resulting in an arteritis and spinal cord ischemia or spinal cord compression secondary to epidural mass effect.

PEARLS:

1. Suspect epidural abscess in the chronically ill or debilitated patient, with local spine pain.

2. WBC, temperature, plain films, and examination may be entirely normal.

3. ESR is elevated in over 90% of these patients.

4. Myelogram is the most sensitive radiological test to demonstrate epidural abscess.

5. Treatment is based on early diagnosis, prompt administration of antibiotics, and surgical decompression.

6. Where surgical decompression is not warranted, confirmation of organism type and sensitivity can be made by Craig needle biopsy of the disc space or vertebral body.

PITFALLS:

1. <u>Failure to promptly diagnose epidural abscess may lead to irreversible neurological deficits</u>.

2. Multiple organisms may be present and should be considered particularly in the patient who is not responding to medical management.

3. Associated sources of infection, if they are not identified and treated, may continue to seed and act as a source of recurrent infection.

4. Spinal tap may drain the abscess cavity and this must be appreciated to prevent intradural spread of infection. Lumbar punctures must be performed with care.

REFERENCES

1. Allen MB, Beveridge WD: Spinal epidural and subdural abscesses. In Wilkins RH, Rengachy SS, eds. Neurosurgery. New York, McGraw-Hill, 1985, pp 1972-1975.

2. Baker AS, Ojemann RG, Swartz MN, Richardson EP: Spinal epidural abscess. N Engl J Med 293:463-468, 1975.

3. Danner RL, Hartmen BJ: Update of spinal epidural abscess: 35 cases and review of the literature. Rev Inf Diseases 9:265-274, 1987.

4. Feldenzer JA, McKeever PE, Schaberg DR, Campbell JA, Hoff JT: Experimental spinal epidural abscess: a pathophysiological model in the rabbit. Neurosurgery 20:859-867, 1987.

CHILD WITH PROGRESSIVE BRAIN STEM SIGNS

CASE 39: An 8-year-old girl presents with a 3-month history of change in personality, irritability and decreasing academic performance in school. The mother has also noted increasing stumbling and clumsiness with the right hand. More recently the right eye appeared to turn inward and the child began walking with her head turned to one side. When the child awakened one morning with a drooping on the right side of the face, her parents sought medical assistance.

Admission neurological examination revealed a pleasant, awake, alert child. Pupils were equally round and reactive. There was a right VIth nerve palsy with failure of abduction of the right eye. There was loss of sensation over the right face. There was a right facial paralysis, but cranial nerves VIII through XII were intact. There were increased reflexes on the left side with an upgoing toe. There was evidence of right dysmetria and gait ataxia.

Neuroradiological studies revealed an asymmetrically enlarged pons with irregular borders. The mesencephalic and pontine cisterns were compressed. The ventricular system was not dilated. There was an exophytic component to the tumor and it was irregularly enhancing. The magnetic resonance imaging (MRI) scan (T_2 weighted image) revealed edema throughout the pons with a small central necrotic portion to the tumor, which was centered in the right pons. (See Fig. 39.1 on next page.)

Neuroanatomical Clue:

Understanding the various nuclei of the brain stem and in this case the pons, helps to localize the lesion. The clinical picture can be explained by understanding the anatomy of the pons. (See Fig. 39.2 on next page.)

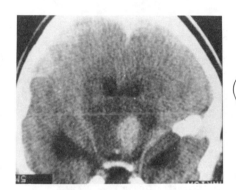

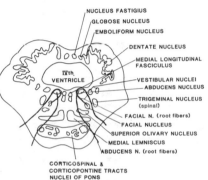

NUCLEUS FASTIGIUS
GLOBOSE NUCLEUS
EMBOLIFORM NUCLEUS
DENTATE NUCLEUS
MEDIAL LONGITUDINAL FASCICULUS
IVth. VENTRICLE
VESTIBULAR NUCLEI
ABDUCENS NUCLEUS
TRIGEMINAL NUCLEUS (spinal)
FACIAL N. (root fibers)
FACIAL NUCLEUS
SUPERIOR OLIVARY NUCLEUS
MEDIAL LEMNISCUS
ABDUCENS N. (root fibers)
CORTICOSPINAL & CORTICOPONTINE TRACTS
NUCLEI OF PONS

Figure 39.1   Figure 39.2

QUESTIONS:

1. What is the most likely diagnosis? What other posterior fossa tumors are seen in childhood?

2. Describe the structures within the pons and their correlation with the symptoms seen in this child.

3. Describe the various neuroradiological studies which might be used to establish this diagnosis?

4. Describe treatment modalities and outcome as seen with this tumor.

ANSWERS:

1. When a young child presents with multiple cranial
    nerve palsies, particularly VIth and VIIth nerve
    palsies, brain stem glioma is the most likely
    diagnosis. Differential diagnosis of brain stem
    gliomas includes extraaxial tumors which may mimic
    them clinically but can usually be distinguished
    radiologically and include medulloblastomas,
    cerebellar astrocytomas, ependymomas,
    hemangioblastomas, and chordomas. Rarely focal
    encephalitis, infection, arteriovenous
    malformations, and epidermoids may mimic brain stem
    gliomas.

2. Brain stem gliomas often start in the region of the
    VIth and VIIth nerve nuclei (see Fig. 39.2). The
    VIth and VIIth nerve palsy seen in this child are
    the result of involvement of these nuclei by tumor.
    Motor symptoms are seen late in the progression of
    brain stem gliomas and are caused by involvement of
    the corticospinal tract. Corticospinal fibers
    originate in the motor cortex and descend into the
    midbrain cerebral peduncles. Fibers carrying
    information to the leg are lateral and fibers to
    the arm are medial. At the pons, these pathways
    are broken up into a series of bundles which come
    together again at the lower pons. In the medulla
    they decussate, again arm fibers are medial and
    cross above the more lateral leg fibers. The arm
    fibers also assume the medial position in the
    corticospinal tract within the opposite side of the
    spinal cord. Sensory pathways seem extremely
    resistant to infiltration by tumor and many
    patients die of their tumors without any signs of
    sensory loss. Cerebellar signs can be seen with
    pontine gliomas either because of compression of
    the cerebellum or involvement of the superior
    cerebellar peduncle. This causes ipsilateral
    ataxia.

3. Computerized tomography has replaced
    pneumoencephalography in diagnosing lesions of the
    brain stem. Correct computed tomography (CT)
    detection is now greater than 95% for brain stem

lesions. Metrizamide cisternography is a useful
adjunct in delineating exophytic extensions of
these tumors.

More recently, the development of MRI has
revolutionized the evaluation and follow up of
patients with brain stem gliomas. The various
sectional planes available (sagittal, coronal, and
axial) give a much better appreciation of the three
dimensional shape of these tumors. Where
available, MRI is the single most valuable study in
evaluating brain stem lesions.

Angiography is reserved for those lesions which
may be vascular, such as arteriovenous
malformations or hemangioblastomas.

4. Surgical intervention for brain stem gliomas is a
   controversial subject. When the tumor extends into
   the fourth ventricle or has a significant exophytic
   or cystic component, surgery may be beneficial.
   Tumors located at the cervical medullary junction
   are usually low grade gliomas and are often
   improved with surgery.

   Tumors in the more rostral aspects of the brain
   stem are usually malignant and although surgery may
   assist with a definitive diagnosis, these tumors
   cannot be completely removed. Biopsy may be
   sufficient for providing a tissue diagnosis but
   because of histological variation within this
   tumor, sampling errors may occur.

   Radiation therapy is the favored form of
   treatment. It is of benefit in 80-90% of patients,
   particularly those with low grade gliomas. In
   surgically inaccessible lesions, radiation therapy
   may be elected without biopsy.

   Survival rates vary with tumor histology. Five
   year survival rates after irradiation vary from 15
   to 40%. In malignant gliomas, untreated survival
   was 2.7 months versus 6.3 months with radiation.
   With benign astrocytomas, children averaged a
   survival of 32.4 months after diagnosis.

Those patients whose brain stem gliomas present with cranial nerve findings, showing diffuse tumor on CT and mitoses on histology, have a much poorer prognosis. Children with CT-enhancing low grade tumors that contain calcifications and Rosenthal fibers on histology are effectively treated with radiation and have a slightly better prognosis. More recently multidrug chemotherapy has been tried with early reports showing some success.

PEARLS:

1. Brain stem gliomas are common childhood tumors and account for 10 to 25% of all intracranial childhood tumors. More recently brain stem gliomas have been classified on the basis of location, intrinsic or extrinsic to the brain stem, enhancement, and presence of solid or cystic components. These factors help in making the diagnosis and in predicting survival rates.

2. Histologically brain stem gliomas range from low grade (grade I or II) astrocytomas to more malignant tumors (grade III or IV, or glioblastoma multiforme). At autopsy approximately 60-70% of brain stem gliomas exhibit foci of hemorrhage, necrosis, and variable degrees of pleomorphism. Radiological evidence of hemorrhage, necrosis, edema and extensive infiltration of the brain stem is correlated with a more malignant tumor histologically.

3. Gliomas of the brain stem have a peak incidence between the ages of 5 to 8 years.

PITFALLS:

1. One of the most characteristic clinical features of brain stem gliomas is the tendency to develop progressive multiple neurological abnormalities without the development of hydrocephalus. The presence of hydrocephalus is not characteristic of brain stem gliomas but can be present.

2. Although generally presenting with bilateral
    symptoms, these tumors may be unilateral with
    significant exophytic components.

3. Accurate history and physical and radiological
    studies are necessary if radiation is elected
    without surgery.

REFERENCES

1. Albright AL, Guthkilch AN, Packer RJ, et al:
    Prognostic factors in pediatric brainstem gliomas. J
    Neurosurg 65:751-755, 1986.

2. Berger MS, Edwards MSB, La Masters D, et al:
    Pediatric brainstem tumors: radiographic,
    pathological and clinical correlations.
    Neurosurgery 12:298-302, 1983.

3. Epstein F, McLeary EL: Intrinsic brainstem tumors of
    childhood surgical indications. J Neurosurg 64:
    11-15, 1986.

4. Fulton DS, Levin VA, Wara WM, et al: Chemotherapy of
    pediatric brainstem tumors. J Neurosurg 54:721-
    725, 1981.

5. Stronik AR, Hoffman HJ, Hendrick EB, Humphreys RP:
    Diagnosis and management of pediatric brainstem
    gliomas. Neurosurgery 65:745-750, 1986.

NEWBORN CHILD WITH LUMBAR DEFECT

<u>CASE 40</u>: This 4.2-kg male child was the product of a
full term uncomplicated pregnancy and was born to a
gravida one, para one 28-year-old mother in excellent
health, with an unremarkable family history.

At birth, the child was noted to have excellent
Apgar scores with stable vital signs. Head circumference was
2 standard deviations above normal for age. The
anterior fontanelle was soft with good pulsations.

Examination of the lumbosacral region revealed a
large reddened weeping sac, 6 cm wide and located at
the L3 region. Through the sac could be seen a large
neural placode. The sac was actively draining
cerebrospinal fluid (CSF).

Neurologically the child had intact cranial nerves
with an excellent suck. Upper extremities were strong
with a good grasp. There was no movement at the ankles
and the feet were inverted with marked equinovarus.
Reflexes were decreased at both ankles. There was no
anal wink. Plain films revealed a spina bifida from
the sacrum to L2.

Ultrasonogram of the head showed moderate
ventricular dilation with a rounded third ventricle.
Computed tomography (CT) scan of the head showed
ventricular enlargement. Cerebellar tonsils were at
the level of the foramen magnum. CT scan of the spine
showed bifid elements from L2 to the sacrum with poorly
formed posterior arches from L4 to the sacrum. The end
of the spinal cord (conus) was located at the level of
the myelomeningocele and the sac could be seen to
contain neural elements.
(See Fig. 40.1 on next page.)

<u>Clue</u>: Important to understanding midline neural tube
defects is an appreciation of the different terms and
their definitions.

<u>Meningocele</u> - consists only of a spinal fluid filled
sac with meningeal and cutaneous coverings. It
contains no spinal or neural elements. True
meningoceles are rare.

<u>Myelomeningocele</u> - consists of herniation of neural
tissue through a defect in bony elements of the spine.
It is covered by imperfect dermal elements and
generally leaks   CSF.   Dura and arachnoid are often
exposed and open to the air.

<u>Lipomyelomeningocele</u> - has all of the elements of a
true myelomeningocele as well as a significant fatty
tissue component.

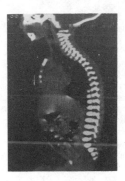

Figure 40.1

QUESTIONS:

1. Describe the embryology of the spinal cord and the
   defect found in myelomeningocele?

2. What are the treatment alternatives for this child?

3. What is the surgical approach to repair of the
   myelomeningocele?

4. What associated medical problems should be
   identified during the immediate management of this
   child?

5. What long term problems might be expected for this
   child?

6. What advice might you offer these parents regarding
   future children?

ANSWERS:

1.   The central nervous system begins as a focal
     proliferation of ectoderm. A central groove
     develops and forms two folds of neural tissue. At
     approximately gestational day 20-28 the lips of
     this fold touch and the tube fuses. The fusion
     starts at the center to eventually become the
     craniovertebral junction. This fusion proceeds in
     a caudal and cephalic direction; the caudal section
     is the last to close. A plane develops between the
     neural ectoderm which has fused and the overlying
     superficial ectoderm. Between these layers migrate
     mesenchymal cells. These mesenchymal cells give
     rise to the arch of the vertebrae and the
     paraspinal muscles. Two major causes have been
     offered to explain myelomeningocele. The first
     theorizes that there is a failure to close of the
     neural tube. The second hypothesizes that in utero
     hydrocephalus causes a blow out of the already
     closed neural tube thus causing the
     myelomeningocele.

2.   Ethical issues regarding management alternatives in
     myelomeningocele are beyond the scope of this
     monograph. Few, if any, chronic care institutions
     will accept a child with an open myelomeningocele
     and untreated hydrocephalus. Therefore full and
     aggressive treatment is extended to all children
     except those in an already agonal, severely
     disabled state at birth.

        Management plans for such a child start in the
     delivery room and require a multi-disciplinary
     approach which involves pediatric, neurosurgical,
     orthopedic, and urological care. Once the decision
     has been made to treat such a child, surgical
     closure of the myelomeningocele must be performed
     in a timely fashion. Delayed closure of the
     myelomeningocele causes and increase in infection
     and in some studies a decrease in motor function.
     The goal of all intervention is to preserve
     existing neural tissue. The child must be kept on
     his abdomen and the sac must not be allowed to dry.
     It should be covered with nonadherent dressings

moistened with normal saline. Antimicrobial agents
and solutions containing iodine should not be used
as they cause damage to neural tissue.

In examining a child with myelomeningocele,
motor and sensory levels are related to the
anatomical level of the lesion but there may be
some preserved function below this level.
Asymmetry of the examination must raise the
possibility of diastematomyelia or other anomaly.
A single midline fusion defect may be associated
with defects at other levels, and therefore,
further evaluation including CT, myelogram, and
magnetic resonance imaging (MRI) may be necessary.

3. <u>Surgical management of the open myelomeningocele
    involves reestablishment of the neural canal</u>. As
    with all congenital anomalies initial dissection
    involves identification of normal planes.

The goal of this dissection is to establish the
pia/arachnoid, dural, and fascial planes so that
when completed the neural placode is free, floating
in CSF, and covered by arachnoid, dura, and well
formed dermal elements. Such repairs may be
particularly difficult in the thoracic and upper
lumbar areas because of associated kyphotic
deformity. Plastic reconstructive surgery may be
necessary with pedicle grafts used to close a large
skin defect. Cosmesis, although a consideration,
is not the major goal of such surgery.

Postoperatively the child should be maintained
either on the side or the abdomen to prevent damage
of the repair. Careful attention to maintenance of
a clean, dry dressing is necessary and the wound is
inspected daily for possible leakage of
cerebrospinal fluid or dehiscence.

4. <u>The child with myelomeningocele requires a team
    management approach from the outset and will
    receive continued follow-up for the rest of his or
    her life</u>. The following are among the most common
    problems encountered early on in the management of
    these children.

A. Hydrocephalus - <u>Ninety-eight percent will develop an enlarged ventricular system</u>, with 80-90% requiring a shunting procedure. Shunting is indicated in any child who shows progressive enlargement of the ventricles, increased head circumference, or signs of a Chiari malformation.

B. <u>Chiari II malformation - It has three major elements: cerebellar dysplasia, brain stem displacement, and elongation of the fourth ventricle</u>. Most Chiari II malformations present during the infant years and are the major cause of death in children with myelomeningocele. These children have difficulty with feeding and a weak cry. Episodes of crying may be associated with apnea and a characteristic laryngeal stridor. Prompt evaluation with CT and MRI is necessary. If there is associated hydrocephalus, a shunt may act to ameliorate the symptoms. Posterior fossa decompression may be necessary at an early age in more severe cases.

C. Urinary continence - Intermittent catheterization is probably the single medical advance which has altered the life expectancy and quality of life for children with myelomeningocele. Using catheterization and pharmacotherapy, urinary continence now approaches 80-90% in such children as they reach adolescence. Rarely are urinary diversion procedures necessary and with careful attention to catheterization technique, infections can be kept to a minimum. It is important to be certain that the bladder is being emptied completely and later in life baseline and follow-up urodynamics will be necessary.

D. Orthopedic problems - Multiple orthopedic procedures are usually necessary. These children may require corrective procedures for their kyphosis, scoliosis, hip abnormalities, and multiple foot deformities. Early orthopedic evaluation is essential so that well planned follow-up can be made.

5. Later deterioration in children with myelomeningocele is uncommon and must be evaluated

aggressively with somatosensory evoked potentials, CT, myelography, and MRI when appropriate. <u>Shunt malfunction, tethered cord, inclusion epidermoid tumors, diastematomyelia, progressive scoliosis, development of orthopedic problems to hip, knee and ankle; and late onset of Chiari II malformations symptoms may all develop in later years</u>. All are amenable to surgical intervention and must be identified in a timely fashion.

Children with myelomeningocele may require special education to reach their full potential. Recent studies suggest that there is not a significant difference in intelligence quotient (IQ) in children with myelomeningocele and the normal population with a single exception. Children who have been shunted and have developed a postoperative infection have lower intelligence. Mean IQ for the normal population is 100, for children with myelomengocel 102, for those shunted but without infection 95, and for those shunted but with infection 73.   Prevention of meningitis and shunt infection is a major goal in managing these children.

Ambulation is possible in 80-90% of these children and is particularly high among children with low lumbar or sacral myelomeningoceles.   Most thoracic meningoceles will not be ambulatory as adults and will be wheelchair bound.

These children require attention to physical therapy early on as contractures and failure to adequately brace can lead to unnecessary morbidity. Again, long-term consistent and coordinated follow-up is essential in these cases.

6. The causes of myelomeningocele are still unknown but genetic factors are believed to be important. <u>The risk to the general population is 1-2 per 1000 births in the United States</u>.   In families who have already had one child afflicted the risk increases to 2.5%.   There are some recent British studies which suggest that administration of vitamins and folic acid supplements markedly reduces the expected rate of neural tube defects in families with children with myelomeningocele.   These

observations have not been confirmed by other observers.

Alpha-fetoprotein (AFP) is a protein which is present in fetal tissue. It is released into amniotic fluid until the anterior abdominal wall and the posterior neural tube close. It will remain increased in amniotic fluid if either remains open and will be increased in maternal blood as well. Mothers with a previous child with a neural tube defect or strong family history or mothers with two serum samples with elevated AFP should have amniocentesis and fetal ultrasound to more accurately assess whether the fetus has myelomeningocele.

PEARLS:

1. Children with myelomeningocele require early aggressive management by a team of trained professionals within 24-48 hours of birth.

2. Hydrocephalus is an important early feature which must be identified and managed.

3. Normal intelligence is possible in 70-75% of these children.

4. Myelomeningocele is a lifelong disease requiring lifelong monitoring on many levels.

PITFALLS:

1. Central nervous system infection is an important cause of mental retardation in this population.

2. Chiari II malformation is a significant cause of morbidity and must be identified early on.

3. Deterioration of neurological function requires aggressive evaluation and treatment.

4. Selection criteria for those to be operated upon is of limited value and is often impossible to employ because of placement problems for such children in chronic care facilities.

REFERENCES

1. Ames MD, Schut L: Results of treatment of 171
   consecutive myelomeningoceles 1963 to 1968.
   Pediatrics 50 466-470, 1972.

2. Carmel PW: The Chiaria malformations and
   syringomyelia.   In Hoffman HJ, Epstein F, eds:
   Disorders of the developing nervous system:
   diagnosis and treatment.   Blackwell Scientific
   Publication, Boston, 1986, pp 133-151.

3. French BN: Midline fusion defects and defects of
   formation. In Youmans JR, ed. Neurological surgery
   Saunders Co, Philadelphia, 1982, pp 1236-1380.

4. Hoffman HJ, Hendrick EB, Humphreys RP: The tethered
   spinal cord: its protean manifestations, diagnosis
   and surgical correction.   Child's Brain 2:145-155,
   1976.

5. Lorber J, Salfiedl S: Results of selective
   treatment of spina bifida cystica. Arch Dis Child
   56:822-830, 1981.

6. McLone DG: Techniques for closure of
   myelomeningocele.   Child's Brain 6:65-73, 1980.

7. Reigel DH: Spina bifida. In Pediatric neurosurgery.
   New York, Grune & Stratton, Inc. 1982, pp 23-
   47.

8. Soare P, Raimondi AJ: Intellectual and perceptual-
   motor characteristics of treated myelomeningocele
   children.   Am J Dis Child 131:199-204, 1977.

54-YEAR-OLD MAN WITH INTERMITTENT LOW BACK PAIN

CASE 41: A 54-year-old man in otherwise good health presented with a 5-year history of low back pain of moderate severity. Over the past 6 months the patient noticed pain eminating from the right buttock down the left lower extremity laterally into the foot. The pain was sharp and deep in quality and occurred when the patient was standing for a long period of time or walked more than two blocks. Often the pain was associated with an unpleasant tingling sensation on the lateral aspect of the foot. Infrequently he experienced right lower extremity pain of a similar quality but of less intensity. The patient's symptoms were relieved by sitting or leaning against a wall with some flexion at the hips and knees, or by lying down.

The patient denied any lower extremity weakness but stated that often the left foot felt clumsy when walking because of the associated pain. He denied bowel or bladder symptoms.

Physical examination including neurological examination was unremarkable. In particular there was no spinal tenderness and straight leg raising was negative.

Computed tomography (CT) scans of the lumbar spine showed hypertrophic changes of the facet joints (see Fig. 41.1).

Figure 41.1:

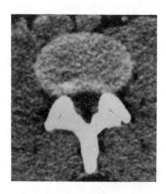

QUESTIONS:

1. At this point two important diagnostic
   possibilities must be considered. What are they and
   what are the elements of the history and physical
   examination that help to distinguish between the
   two?

2. What radiological studies would you order next to
   confirm your diagnosis?

3. Describe the anatomical changes associated with
   lumbar spinal stenosis.

4. Although in most patients with spinal stenosis the
   disorder is degenerative in origin and occurs in
   late middle age, there are subgroups of patients in
   which the disease is congenital or part of a
   systemic disease process. Describe examples of
   these subgroups of patients.

ANSWERS:

1. This patient presents with intermittent lower extremity pain exacerbated by walking. The two diagnoses which must be considered are intermittent claudication due to vascular insufficiency and intermittent neurogenic claudication. The histories may appear quite similar but certain elements may be used to differentiate the two.

    In intermittent claudication from vascular insufficiency the pain is typically burning and cramp-like, affecting both the calf and the thigh muscles. It is relieved by rest and usually occurs in patients with risk factors for peripheral vascular disease such as hypertension and smoking. Intermittent neurogenic claudication is different in that the pain can often be elicited by standing and is relieved with recumbency or, as in this patient, by standing against a wall with the hips and knees flexed. There is usually associated back pain.

    The physical examination as in this patient may be quite normal. It is often necessary to observe the patient's walk or carefully hyperextend the spine in order to elicit the patient's symptoms. One must be alert to the signs of peripheral vascular disease such as diminished peripheral pulses and trophic skin changes including lack of hair over the legs.

    It is obvious that by history and physical examination alone one cannot always distinguish between intermittent neurogenic claudication and claudication secondary to peripheral vascular disease. For this reason additional examinations are often necessary, including noninvasive Doppler flow studies or femoral angiography should a vascular etiology be suspected.

2. Because this patient's history is rather classic for intermittent neurogenic claudication, evaluation should then be directed at the lumbar spine. Computed tomography (CT) scanning is particularly helpful in this regard as it can demonstrate the dimensions of the spinal canal in cross section.

Myelography is useful in delineating the course of
the nerve roots and should be performed when
surgery is contemplated.

3. In spinal stenosis <u>the sagittal diameter of the</u>
    <u>spinal canal is reduced as are the dimensions of</u>
    <u>the lateral recesses and foramens of the nerve</u>
    <u>roots</u>. This is usually the result of degenerative
    changes in the spine including hypertrophied facet
    joints and the formation of spondylotic bars
    anterior to the spinal canal. In addition,
    thickening of the ligamentum flavum helps to
    decrease the transverse diameter of the spinal
    canal. The process may be segmental or generalized
    and in up to 15% of patients is associated with
    symptomatic cervical spondylosis or cervical
    stenosis.

    Often the lateral recess is narrowed out of
    proportion to the rest of the spinal canal. This
    characteristically results in radicular symptoms as
    noted in this patient.

    It is important to note that in patients with
    spinal stenosis, <u>disc herniation of an otherwise</u>
    <u>minor degree may result in significant nerve root</u>
    <u>compresssion</u> and symptoms as the spinal canal is
    already compromised by the bony hypertrophy.

    Surgery is aimed at decompressing the thecal sac
    and involved nerve roots by removing the overlying
    bone posteriorly. Laminectomy with foramenotomy
    and removal of portions of the bony facet joint are
    usually performed depending on the location of the
    stenosis.

4. <u>Achondroplasia represents a classic example of</u>
    <u>congenital spinal stenosis</u>. This is an autosomal
    dominant disease in which there is a decrease of
    endochondral bone formation at the growth plate and
    a resultant premature closure of the epiphyses.
    The spine is usually normal in length but the
    lamina are thick and the pedicles short thus
    narrowing the sagittal dimension of the spinal
    canal. The stenosis is generalized throughout the
    spine and symptoms occur due to cord and/or nerve
    root compression.

Spinal stenosis may also occur as a finding in acromegaly. In this case <u>excessive growth hormone secreted by a pituitary tumor results in bony overgrowth and spinal stenosis</u>. In Paget's disease there is rapid bone resorption followed by formation of architecturally and chemically abnormal bone.

<u>Spinal stenosis occurs in some patients with Paget's disease and can be successfully treated with decompressive laminectomy</u>. The bone in these cases is highly vascular and the surgeon must pay careful attention to hemostasis.

PEARLS:

1. In the initial evaluation of the patient with lower extremity pain exacerbated by walking always keep in mind the diagnoses of intermittent neurogenic claudication <u>and</u> intermittent claudication due to vascular insufficiency.

2. The presence of an acutely herniated disc in an elderly patient with lumbar stenosis is an uncommon finding.

PITFALLS:

1. <u>Patients with lumbar stenosis frequently have coexisting cervical stenosis</u>. Care must be taken in manipulating the cervical spine in these patients particularly under general anesthesia.

2. Advanced age is not a contradiction for surgery in the treatment of lumbar stenosis as excellent results are frequently obtained in these age groups.

REFERENCES

1. Evans JG: Neurogenic intermittent claudication. Br Med J 2:985-987, 1964.

2. Ray CD: New techniques for decompression of lumbar spinal stenosis. Neurosurgery 10:587-592, 1982.

PATIENT WITH PROGRESSIVE HAND WEAKNESS AND NUMBNESS

CASE 42: A 39-year-old man presented with gradual onset of neck pain, hand weakness, and numbness over a 2-year period. His past history was remarkable for an auto accident 5 years ago. At that time he suffered a loss of consciousness and a transient loss of upper extremity strength which gradually resolved over several weeks. In addition he had several long bone fractures.

Recently he had noticed difficulty manipulating fine objects, and he had burned himself accidentally, being unaware that he was touching a hot object. He also noted increasing neck pain radiating to both shoulders. Pain and sensory changes worsened with straining or coughing.

His neurological examination was remarkable for normal mentation, intact cranial nerves, and normal cerebellar function. There was bilateral weakness of both upper extremities, loss of tendon reflexes in the upper extremities, with increased reflexes in the lower extremities. There was bilateral loss of pain and temperature over the shoulders, arms, hand, and chest. His hand muscles were atrophic, worse on the right than left, and he walked with a spastic gait.

Clue: Saggital magnetic resonance imaging (MRI) of the spine revealed an intramedullary cyst from C3 to T4 (see next page).

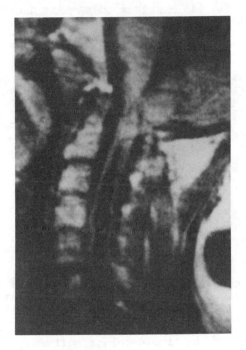

Figure 42.1

QUESTIONS:

1. What is this patient's diagnosis? What is the
   pathophysiology of the patient's presenting
   symptoms?

2. What are the causes and associated anomalies seen
   with this lesion?

3. What radiological studies might be useful?

4. What are the treatment options for this patient?

ANSWERS:

1. <u>Syringomyelia - This condition is a cavitation
    within the spinal cord resulting in central cord
    destruction</u>. The deficits appreciated are readily
    explained by the associated structures which are
    destroyed or compressed.

    The location of this lesion interrupts the
    lateral spinothalamic fibers which decussate
    centrally within the spinal cord. Because these
    fibers conduct pain and temperature to the upper
    extremity, this results in a loss of pain and
    temperature in a cape-like distribution over both
    sides of the body. There is no sensory impairment
    in the lower extremities. Proprioception and touch
    are maintained in the upper extremities. This
    cape-like distribution of selective sensory
    modality loss is characteristic of the sensory
    disassociation seen with syringomyelia. As the
    disease progresses, the anterior gray horns are
    compressed resulting in atrophy in the hand mucles.
    Eventually there are signs of pyramidal tract
    damage with resulting increase in lower extermity
    reflexes.

2. Many causes of syringomyelia have been hy
    pothesized. It can be idiopathic, without any
    other associated abnormality or precipitating
    event. It can be seen with obstruction of the
    foramen magnum and dilation of the central canal as
    seen with the Arnold-Chiari malformation.
    <u>Syringomyelia can be associated with spinal cord
    tumors, secondary to trauma with resulting
    intramedullary hemorrhage, associated with vascular
    anomalies of the spine, and may be seen in severe
    spinal arachnoiditis</u>.

3. The neuroradiological picture and examination
    clearly characterize syringomyelia. Metrizimide
    myelography and delayed computed tomography (CT)
    usually demonstrate the syrinx as contrast material
    fills the cavity. The sagittal view afforded by
    the MRI helps delineate the extent of such lesions.
    A syrinx appears black on T1 weighted images and
    white on T_2 weighted images.

4. Decompressing the syrinx cavity is the goal of any
    of the therapeutic modalities. When a source for
    the syrinx can be identified, treatment is
    accordingly directed. Chiari malformations are
    decompressed and intramedullary tumors are removed.
    The isolated syrinx is decompressed by shunting the
    cavity. Such shunts can be connected from the
    syrinx cavity to the subarachnoid space within the
    spinal canal, to the pleural space, and to the
    peritoneum. The natural history of patients with
    syringomyelia is one of gradual loss of
    neurological function over many years. Most series
    report a 20-50% progression of symptoms in patients
    who have initially responded to surgical
    decompression. Many benefit from repeated shunting
    procedures.

PEARLS:

1. Differential diagnosis of syringomyelia includes
    Chiari Type I malformation in which there is
    extension of the cerebellar tonsil below the
    foramen magnum resulting in dilation of the central
    canal. It is associated with nystagmus, cerebellar
    ataxia (truncal greater than appendicular),
    exertional head and neck pain, and hydrocephalus.
    Intramedullary spinal cord tumors may cause
    symptoms which resemble syringomyelia by virtue of
    the tracts that are involved. Such tumors include
    astrocytomas, ependymomas and less likely
    metastatic tumors. Hemangioblastomas are often
    associated with cystic components.

2. In posttraumatic cases there is an associated
    central area of necrosis and hemorrhage which later
    goes on to create a cystic cavity within the cord.
    Arteriovenous malformations and other vascular
    anomalies may also hemorrhage into the cord and
    result in cystic cavities.

PITFALLS:

1. It is unfortunate, but diversionary procedures are often effective only for a short time. The natural history of syringomyelia is one of progressive neurological deterioration.

2. It is important to define associated anomalies, particularly Chiari malformation as these are amenable to other forms of treatment.

REFERENCES

1. Aubin ML, Vignaud J, Jardin C, Bar D: Computed tomography in 75 clinical cases of syringomyelia. AJNR 2:199-204, 1981.

2. Faulhauer K, Leow K; The surgical treatment of syringomyelia: long-term results. Acta Neurochir (Wein) 44:215-222, 1978.

3. Krayenbuhl H: Evaluation of the different surgical approaches in the treatment of syringomyelia. Clin Neurol Neurosurg 77:110-118, 1974.

4. Newman PK, Terenty TR, Foster JB: Some observations on the pathogenesis of syringomyelia. J. Neurol Neurosurg Psych 44:964-969, 1981.

5. Schlesinger EB, Antunes JL, Michelsen WJ, Louis KM: Hydromyelia: clinical presentation and comparison of modialities of treatment. Neurosurgery 9:356-365, 1981.

6. Williams B: On the pathogenesis of syringomyelia. A review. J R Soc Med 73:798-806, 1980.

Index

Anisocoria, 92
Anticoagulation, 82, 138
Anticonvulsants, 30, 115
Antifibrinolytic agents, 16
Antiplatelet agents, 210
Aqueductal stenosis, 20
Arachnoid cyst, 57
Arachnoiditis, fibrosing, 20
Arm
  pain, in cervical spondylosis, 40-41
  weakness with loss of sensation in leg,
    6-11
Arnold-Chiari malformations
  associated disorders, 145-146
  diagnosis of, 143, 144
  magnetic resonance imaging, 143
  normal pressure hydrocephalus and,
    20
  surgical decompression, 145, 249
  syringomyelia and, 248, 250
  type II, with myelomeningocele, 236,
    238
  types, 145
Arteriography, 144
Arteriovenous fistulas, 95
Arteriovenous malformations
  age and, 109-110
  angiography, 200, 229
  autoregulation of cerebral vascular
    system, 112
  clinical presentation, 34, 109
  cryptic, 111
  diagnosis of, 108
  differential diagnosis, 228
  intracerebellar bleeding and, 82, 83
  intracerebral hemorrhage and, 189,
    191
  location, 111
  of spinal cord
    angiogram, 44, 45
    cutaneous vascular anomalies, 49
    prognosis, 50
    treatment, 48-49
    types, 47-48
  proptosis and, 34
  surgical decision making, 110
  treatment, 110
Arteritis, 105
Aspirin, for transient ischemic attack,
  210

Astrocytomas
  calcium deposits in, 78
  cerebellar, 228
  cystic cerebellar, 78
  diagnosis of, 27, 29
  glial cell tumors and, 121
  grade IV, 76
  histologic classification, 120
  in posterior fossa, 214
  incidence of, 8
  location of, 79
  progression of, 79
  projection into ventricles, 133
  subependymal, 214
Ataxia, ipsilateral appendicular, 82
Atlantoocipital fusion, 144
Auditory nerve, 4
Aura, 26

Basilar artery aneurysm, 105
Basilar impression, 144
Batson's plexus, 129, 164
Beta human chorionic gonadotropin, 121
Birth control pills, pseudotumor cerebri
  and, 72
Birth trauma, 146
Blacks, hypertension and, 188
Blindness, transient monocular, 208
Blood dyscrasias, 105
Bone scans, of epidural mass, 223
Bony tumors, 98
Brachalgia, 41
Brachycephaly, 182
Brain
  injury determination from gunshot
    wound, 92-93
  metastases, 165
  vascular malformations, 108
Brain stem auditory evoked responses
  (BAERs), 3
Brain stem gliomas
  clinical features, 230-231
  histologic grading, 230
  incidence, 230
  motor symptoms, 228
  prognosis, 229-230
  radiation therapy, 229
  surgical treatment, 229
Brain stem infarction, 83
Brain stem signs, progressive, 226-231
Brain tumors (see also specific tumors)

252

extraneural metastasis, 78
incidence, 216
mixed primary, 79
Breast cancer metastases, 126, 164-166
Brown-S;aaequard syndrome, 46
Burst fracture, cervical, 60
"Butterfly glioma," 78

Caf;aae au lait spots, with proptosis and
decreased visual acuity, 32-36
Calcium channel blockers, 16
Calcium deposits
giant aneurysms and, 68
in suprasellar region, 98
in temporal lobe mass, 25
tumors associated with, 78
Calvarium, development of, 182
Cancer (see also specific cancers)
central nervous system involvement,
165
Caroticocavernous fistula, 34, 202-204
Carotid artery
aneurysms of, 57
proximal internal, aneurysm, 66
puncture, 160
Carotid bruits, 211
Carotid cavernous fistula
differential diagnosis, 204
etiology, 202
spontaneous, 204
symptoms and diagnosis, 34, 202-203
Carotid endarterectomy, 210-211
Cauda equina compression, 172
Cauda equina syndrome, 178, 180
Caudal medulla, intramedullary mass
lesion, 6
Cavernous hemangiomas, 8
Cavernous malformations, 108, 109, 189
Cavernous sinus, 201
Cavernous sinus thrombosis, 67, 204
Central nervous system
as metastases site, 165
development, 234
Central venous pressure, 16
Cerebellar astrocytomas, 228
Cerebellar cysts, 199
Cerebellar hemangioblastomas, 198, 200
Cerebellar hematomas, 84
Cerebellar infarction, 83
Cerebellopontine angle
nerves of, 2, 4

tumor, 159
Cerebral arteries, anterior and middle,
104
Cerebral edema, 116
Cerebritis, from radiotherapy, 79
Cerebrospinal fluid
parameningeal infectious process,
222-223
pressure in normal pressure
hydrocephalus, 20-21
tumor seeding, 122-123, 134
Cervical bruits, 211, 212
Cervical canal, sagittal diameter
narrowing, 38, 40
Cervical spine injury
burst or compression fracture, 60
emergency management, 61-62
fracture, 116
immobilization, 42
indications for cervical traction, 60
lower, 62
prevertebral soft tissue space, 270
severity, 62
suspicion of, 58
upper, 62
Cervical spondylosis
clinical triad, 40-41
location, 42
neck, excessive manipulation of, 43
treatment, 42
Cervical traction, 42, 60, 61
Chemodectoma, 120
Chemotherapy
for glioblastoma, 77
for pineal region tumors, 122
Chiari malformations (see Arnold-Chiari
malformation)
Chordomas, 67, 98, 228
Choriocarcinoma, 166
Choroid plexus papillomas
diagnosis of, 132, 214
histologic classification, 120
location of, 134
malignant, 134
postoperative complications, 133-134
surgical resection, 133
Chronic pain syndrome, 150-151
Chymopapain, 173-174
Claudication, intermittent neurogenic,
242-243

Drugs (see specific drugs)
Dural sinus injury, 95

Electrocephalography, 3
Electroencephalography, 27
Electromyography, 3
Emboli, from partially thrombosed giant
    aneurysm, 69
Embolization, intravascular, 203
Embryonal cell carcinomas, 120, 121
    (see also specific carcinomas)
Endocrine disorders
    after craniopharyngioma surgery, 101
    pseudotumor cerebri and, 72
    with pineal region tumors, 122
Endodermal sinus tumors, 121
Enhancing vermis, 84
Ependymomas, 8, 120, 198, 214, 228
Epidermoid cysts, 57, 194
Epidermoids, 8, 57, 133, 228
Epidural abscess, 222, 224-225
Epidural hematomas
    craniotomy for, 87
    etiology, 88
    location, 86
    "lucid interval," 87
    posterior fossa, 88
Epidural space, 220
Epidural spinal cord stimulator, 152-153,
    154
Epilepsy
    intractable temporal lobe, 24-30
    risk of chronic subdural hematoma
        and, 138
    surgical treatment, 28-29
Exophthalmos, 204
Eye, pulsation and decreased vision,
    201-204

Facial nerve
    anatomy, 4
    preservation in translabyrinthine
        operation, 2-3
    stimulation, 3
Facial pain, surgical treatment, 156-162
Failed back syndrome, 148-155
Failure to thrive, with increasing head
    size, 131-134
Fistula, carotid cavernous, 34, 202-204
Focal encephalitis, 228
Focal seizure, adult, 75-79

Fontanelles, 182
Foramen magnum herniation, 88
Formen magnum compression
    syndrome, 144
Furosemide, 72

Gait disturbance
    in child, 213-217
    with dementia and urinary
        incontinence, 19-23
    with progressive numbness, 38-43
Galactorrhea, with amenorrhea, 51-57
Gastrointestinal cancer, CNS
    involvement, 165
Generalized tonic-clonic seizures, 24
Germ cell origin tumors, 120
Germinomas, 120, 121, 122
Gigantism, 52
Glasgow Coma Scale, 90, 94, 189
Glial cell tumors, 120
Glioblastomas
    calcium deposits and, 78
    diagnosis of, 76-77
    histologic classification, 120
    location of, 79
    prognosis, 77-78
    surgical treatment, 77
Gliomas
    brain stem (see Brain stem gliomas)
    "butterfly" type, 78
    location of, 57, 194
    malignant, 8
    optic nerve, 34
Gliomatosis cerebri, 79
Gliosis, of spinal cord, radiotherapy, 9
Glomus, malformations, 48
Glycerol, 72
Grand mal seizures, 24
Growth hormone, excessive secretion of,
    244
Growth hormone adenomas, 52
Gunshot wounds in head
    comatose patient and, 95
    in military situations, 95
    mortality rate, 94
    prevention of perioperative infection,
        94
    prognosis, 94-95
    surgical goals, 93-94

H$_2$-antagonists, 94

Hamartoma, 27, 29, 57, 98
Hand, weakness and numbness, 245-*250*
"Harlequin eye" sign, *181*, 183
Head, abnormally shaped of infant,
     181-185
Head trauma
    altered consciousness after, 85-89
    blunt, 58-63
    causing eye pulsation and decreased
         vision, *201*-204
    from gunshot wounds, 90-*95*
    normal pressure hydrocephalus and,
         20
    progressive obtundation after,
         113-116
Headache
    from posterior fossa mass lesion,
         197-200
    from subarachnoid hemorrhage, 106
    normal pressure hydrocephalus and,
         22
    sudden with ataxia, 81-84
    with impaired upgaze, *118*-123
    with midback pain, 44-50
    with nausea, vomiting and stiff neck,
         102-106
    with stiff neck, sudden onset of, 12-17
    with visual loss, 97-101
    with visual obscurations and
         papilledema, 71-74
Hearing loss, with unilateral tinnitus,
     1-5
Hemangioblastomas
    angiography of, 229
    cerebellar, 198, 200
    differential diagnosis, 228
    histologic classification, 120
    incidence of, 8
    location of, 214
    retinal, 198
Hemangiomas, 8, 34
Hemangiopericytomas, 200
Hemanopsias, 138
Hematocrit, 16
Hematomas (*see also* Epidural
         hematomas; Subdural
         hematomas)
    from bullet track, 93
    intracerebellar, 83
Hemianopsia, homonymous, *107*-112

Hemiparesis
    false localizing, 89
    in chronic subdural hematoma, 138
    ipsilateral to IIIrd nerve palsy, 90, 92
Hemiplegia, with intracerebral
         hemorrhage, 186-*191*
Hemorrhage
    cerebellar, 82, 112, 191
    cerebral (*see* Intracerebral
         hemorrhage)
    from arteriovenous malformation, 111
    intratumoral, with cerebellar
         hemangioblastomas, 199
    intraventricular, 133
    subarachnoid (*see* Subarachnoid
         hemorrhage)
Histiocytosis, 34
Hydrocephalus
    communicating, 133, 134
    computed tomography of, 121
    delayed, 17
    etiology, 120
    normal pressure, 20-23
    obstructive, 69, 133, 214
         caused by multi-cystic parasellar
             mass, 192-*196*
         surgical treatment, 195
         with optic nerve glioma, 35, 36
    primary, 133
    secondary, 133
    ventriculoperational shunt, 122
    with choroid plexus papillomas, 133
    with myelomeningocele, 236
Hygromas, 134
Hypernephroma, intracerebral
         hemorrhage and, 189
Hyperosmotic agents, 72
Hyperreflexia, 146
Hypertension
    intracranial, benign, 72-73
    with intracerebral hemorrhage, 188
    with transient neurologic dysfunction,
         206-*212*
Hypoparathyroidism, pseudotumor
         cerebri and, 72
Hypothalamic glioma, 98
Hypothalamus, blood supply of, 100

Impotence, 53
Infarction, cerebellar, 82, 83
Inflammatory conditions, 67